Making a Difference
Stories from the Point of Care
Volume II

BOOKS OF STORIES BY AND ABOUT NURSES

From the Honor Society of Nursing, Sigma Theta Tau International

---

A Daybook for Nurses: Making a Difference Each Day, Hudacek, 2004.

Making a Difference: Stories from the Point of Care, Volume II, Hudacek, 2004.

Pivotal Moments in Nursing: Leaders Who Changed the Path of a Profession, Houser and Player, 2004.

Ordinary People, Extraordinary Lives: The Stories of Nurses, Smeltzer and Vlasses, 2003.

The HeART of Nursing: Expressions of Creative Art in Nursing, Wendler, 2002.

Stories of Family Caregiving: Reconsideration of Theory, Literature, and Life, Poirier and Ayres, 2002.

As We See Ourselves: Jewish Women in Nursing, Benson, 2001.

Cadet Nurse Stories: The Call for and Response of Women During World War II, Perry and Robinson, 2001.

Making a Difference: Stories from the Point of Care, Hudacek, 2000.

The Adventurous Years: Leaders in Action 1973-1999, Watts, 1998.

For more information and to order these and other books from the Honor Society of Nursing, Sigma Theta Tau International, visit **www.nursingsociety.org/publications**; or go to **www.nursingknowledge.org/stti/books**, the Web site of Nursing Knowledge International, the honor society's sales and distribution division; or call 1.888.NKI.4.YOU (U.S. and Canada) or +1.317.634.8171 (outside U.S. and Canada).

Making a Difference
Stories from the Point of Care
Volume II

Sharon Hudacek, RN, EdD

Sigma Theta Tau International
Honor Society of Nursing

Indianapolis, Indiana, USA

Sigma Theta Tau International

Publisher: Jeff Burnham

Acquisitions Editor: Fay L. Bower, RN, DNSc, FAAN

Development Editor: Carla Hall

Proofreaders: Linda Canter, Jane Palmer

Editorial Team: Jennifer Armstrong, Dawn Hamilton, Melody Jones, Mary Ellen Krause, Tonna Thomas

Composition and Interior Design: Rebecca Harmon

Cover Design: Gary Adair

Printed in the United States of America

Printing and Binding by V.G. Reed & Sons

Sigma Theta Tau International

550 West North Street

Indianapolis, IN 46202

Visit our Web site at www.nursingsociety.org/publications for more information on our books and other publications.

ISBN: 1-930538-14-6

Library of Congress Cataloging-in-Publication Data

Hudacek, Sharon.
  Making a difference : stories from the point of care / Sharon Hudacek.
      p. ; cm.
  Volume II.
  ISBN 1-930538-14-6 (pbk.)
  1. Nursing—Anecdotes. 2. Nurse and patient. 3. Caring.
  [DNLM: 1. Nursing—Personal Narratives. 2. Nurse-Patient Relations—Personal Narratives. 3. Nurses—Personal Narratives. 4. Nursing Care—Personal Narratives. WZ 112.5.N8 H883m 2004] I. Title.

RT82.H776 2004
610.73'06'9—dc22

                                                                      2004024575

04 05 06 07 / 9 8 7 6 5 4 3 2 1

I would like to dedicate this book to my husband, Stephen L. Hudacek, and my boys, Stephen and Chas. They have given me the gifts of love, wisdom, generosity, and many precious moments in time.

Acknowledgments

The words of nurses inspired me to write this book—words that are often spoken only by nurses, that are often heard only between nurses. These soft words, tender phrases, and spiritual thoughts are now documented. They are our legacy. They are a part of our profession forever.

I wish to thank so many people who have given me constant support and inspiration, beginning with the wonderful nurses of the Florida Nurses Association: Thanks, sincerely, to all of you for documenting years of clinical exemplars. Your exemplars represent the very best in nursing care. I cherish your work. Thanks to Dr. Francis Smith, Willa Fuller, and Dr. Patricia Quigley for sharing with me the many talents of your nurse colleagues.

To Dr. A. Elaine Bond and my colleagues at Brigham Young University College of Nursing, who contributed to the 50th anniversary celebration called *The Healers Art:* Thank you for sharing your words with me. To Bonnie Wesorick for her writings on nursing leadership; to my research assistants, Mary Bea Maslar and Judith Doherty, for their work in this qualitative project; to Dr. James Pallante, for his support in my research endeavors; to Dr. Patricia Harrington, Dr. Donna Carpenter (best buddy) and colleagues in the Department of Nursing at the University of Scranton; and to Alice Lord and Dawn Mazurik—you really came through for me!

To Elizabeth Kuhns Douglas, for being a creative force and friend: Thanks, Elizabeth, for always seeing the coffee cup as half full! I am entirely grateful for your professionalism and support. To my dear Birthday Club friends—Mar, Stacey, Donna, Kath, Gail, Joanne, and Ro— you are always there, through thick and thin. To my sisters, Kim and

Deb: You are my heroes and give me ambition through your thoughtfulness and caring.

To my mother and father, Kay and Charles Smith: No one could have better parents—ever. You taught me about hard work, because you always worked so hard. Mom, I am grateful for every day that you went to the sewing factory. Dad, every day that you spent in the Pennsylvania mines encouraged all of us to be educated and strong. Your work ethic will never be forgotten. Here's to "The Smith Family."

To Dr. Fay Bower and Jeff Burnham of Sigma Theta Tau International: Thank you for your guidance and encouragement. It is because of you that this book was written. You gave me a chance to be creative in 2000. Four years later, you gave me another chance. I tremendously appreciate it.

Finally, to my husband, Steve, and my sons, Stephen and Chas, who taught me that the greatest pleasure in life is love!

About the Author

Dr. Sharon Hudacek is an associate professor of nursing and director of the LPN to BSN program at the University of Scranton. She is founder of the Making a Difference Foundation, an organization that funds nursing scholarships for LPN students returning for a bachelor's degree in nursing. All *Making a Difference* book profits support this foundation. Her specialty is adult health nursing and pharmacology. She teaches senior nursing students in the three clinical settings at Mercy Hospital Scranton—neuro, orthopedics, and renal—which she considers the most valuable role in her teaching career. The recipient of many honors and awards, she has written *Making a Difference: Stories from the Point of Care,* which won the 2003 Best of Books Award from the Honor Society of Nursing, Sigma Theta Tau International, and *A Daybook for Nurses: Making a Difference Each Day.* Dr. Hudacek is married and lives with her husband, Stephen, and their two sons, Stephen and Chas, in Moosic, Pennsylvania. She is a homeroom and lunchroom mom and a dedicated volunteer for Scranton Prep and Marian Catholic Schools in Scranton, Pennsylvania.

Table of Contents at a Glance

Table of Contents

Preface: A Scrapbook of Stories

"How will the nurses of tomorrow know what it was like to be a nurse in the last quarter of the century?" (Abrams, 1999).

Nursing research has led us to tremendous investigation, objectivity, and validity. But the language of our work, the descriptions of our practice, and the way we inform others can be further expanded through carefully written narratives.

The art of storytelling is a method of teaching, learning, and informing others. The "nurse story" helps us share the skills and emotions involved in caring for patients. Nurses learn that caring is multifaceted and involves complex thinking. The stories in this book help us understand past thinking and decision-making. These stories reveal personal and professional wisdom. It is the story that tells us about the trusting relationship (Leight, 2002). It is the story that assists us in illuminating the practice knowledge we take for granted (Ford & Turner, 2001).

There is renewed attention on the need for nurses, and humans in general, to use narrative analysis. "A narrative framework affords nurse scholars a special access to the human experience of time, order, and change and obligates us to listen to the human impulse to tell tales" (Sandelowski, 1991, p. 165). This need to share the human experience in day-to-day nursing is persuasive and obligatory. It is a way for nurses to reveal the extent of their practice and the magnitude of their caring.

Most importantly, telling stories is a way for nurses to heal. Nurses are now documenting critical memories from their careers. They are drawing from their culture of caring to write descriptions of intense experiences they have undergone. They are ordering past events so they can make sense of them, personally and professionally. Did I do the best I could? Did I make the right decision? Did I advocate for that child in the best way I could? Nurses are socially positioned to talk and write. They are writing, telling, sculpting, and using these and other art forms to heal themselves. As an example of this, my colleague Dianne Duchesne uses story art to depict death, dying, and grief experiences with hospice patients. Her DVD and video portray stories and art she has used to "fully honor the healing relationship." She notes that she has "stumbled on a way to express the very beautiful nature of death, dying, and grief" (D. Duchesne, personal communication, December 2003).

Perhaps few stories have been written in the past because nurses did not believe their experiences were valuable. Behind the scenes, nurses are labeled as silent healthcare partners. Now, however, they see a story in the situation, a tale in the talk, and poetry in the action. Their tears, joys, and emotions are becoming an essential—even vital—reason to write. Transforming their feelings into written narratives may help nurses work more productively and transition more gracefully through their lives and careers.

Nursing is a profession filled with countless stories to tell in many creative ways. Telling the tale heals the nurse's soul. It also ensures that future nurses will know of the greatness of their predecessors' work. It is time to create our scrapbook of stories for present and future generations of nurses.

Introduction

A short time ago, I was visiting a long-term care facility, presenting the Making a Difference in Nursing Award to an outstanding nurse for her work there. Her name is Sandy, a dedicated nurse with tremendous compassion for the elderly. For many residents in this facility, she is their family. For these people, Sandy made their final days memorable by caring for them until the very end.

As I was wending my way past diverse residents in wheelchairs and walkers, I passed many craft rooms, a beautiful chapel, and a trickling waterfall at the exit of the facility. Suddenly, I noticed Chewy, a pug dog, jumping on the lap of one of the residents. Chewy also lives in this facility, along with a Labrador retriever and a host of other pets. The nurses told me that the residents love the animals. They further explained that frequently they try to meet the requests of their ill patients and make the little time they have left on this earth fulfilling. Intrigued, I listened as they shared a story, one that so deeply moved me it sparked my interest, once again, in writing the stories of nurses.

The story goes a bit like this. An elderly patient, let's call him "Ray," was admitted to Mountain View. Like many of the patients, Ray was terminally ill. He was admitted for palliative measures or basically to spend his final days in this facility. Not a social man, Ray lived most of his adult life alone on a farm. He had no family and spoke only of one friend.

He developed a trusting rapport with his nurses and shared with them a secret—actually more a regret than a secret. Throughout his entire life, he had loved songbirds, but he had never had time to take care of one as a pet. His house was always quiet, and if he could live his life over again, he would make sure he bought a songbird. The primary nurse discussed this observation with the director of nursing, which prompted a pleasing adventure. Their quest was to purchase a parakeet and a home for it, to have the bird tested for safety, and then to present it to Ray. The director of nursing approved the expense. Although the bird cost $15, the cage $89, and the testing $125, Ray received his wish. High upon the bedside table the beautiful parakeet, named Ethel, sang to Ray every day and seemed to sing a little louder when Ray's pain grew steadier. The bird helped create relationships between Ray and the staff that were based on trust and understanding. Above all—the hectic pace, beeping monitors, and rolling meal trays—the songbird shared her gift of beauty. In Ray's final moments, the nurses said, the wind blew softly over his face, and his lips curved into a warm, peaceful smile. The nurses watched in awe as the songbird, slowly and ever-so-peacefully, sang to him in his last, tender moments of sleep.

I believe this is not just a story—it is a powerful memory. The example of Ray's care is a transforming experience. It is because of "memories" such as this that I write for nurses. Nurses have tremendous narrative patterns and gripping stories. Etched in the minds of nurses around the world are these compelling accounts of how individual nurses make a difference in the hearts and lives of so many, every day. Countless memories of nurses have not been heard. Until recently, precious few nurse stories have been documented. My worry has always been that our stories will be lost and that future nurses will not learn about the compassionate caring of other nurses. These stories of nurses are our legacy.

The intent of this book is to give nurses a voice and a means by which to document (or journal) their work and caring practices, and allow all of us to reflect upon their stories. These accounts are protected and carefully shared. Writing these stories has, for some, elicited strong feelings, questions, and renewed sorrow. Some anecdotes are joyful, while others are mysterious and tragic. The stories collectively illustrate a deep caring by nurses in all types of settings: long-term care, hospice, schools, and home care. The addition of international nursing stories adds a deeper meaning to this collection and helps to lessen the distance among nurses everywhere. In the chapters that follow, you will read narratives, many of which have never before been shared. These stories, I assure you, are the heart—the essence—of nursing. Follow along as I reveal the beloved stories of nurses who each make a difference in the lives of so many, every day.

(Special thanks to Maryann Rubino, Cara Reed, and the nurses at Mountain View Care Facility in Moosic, Pennsylvania, for the story of Ray and his songbird.)

REFERENCES

Abrams, S.E. (1999). Saving our stories. Public Health Nursing, 16(2), 77-78.

Duchesne, D. (2003). Living on the edge; a story about death, dying and grief (DVD). Available through: Paulo4u@comcast.net.

Ford, K. & Turner, D. (2001). Stories seldom told: Pediatric nurses' experiences of caring for hospitalized children with special needs and their families. Journal of Advanced Nursing, 33(3), 288-295

Leight, S.B. (2002). Starry night: using story to inform aesthetic knowing in women's health nursing. Journal of Advanced Practice, 37(1), 108-114.

Sandelowski, M. (1991). Telling Stories: narrative approaches in qualitative research. Image: Journal of Nursing Scholarship, 23(3), 161-166.

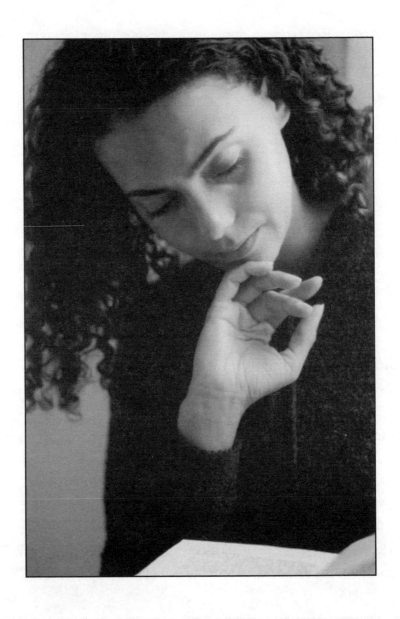

CHAPTER 1

Making a Difference: Nurse Work

Nursing is an art; and if it is to be made an art, it requires as exclusive a devotion, as hard a preparation, as any painter's or sculptor's work; for what is the having to do with dead canvas or cold marble, compared with having to do with the living body— the temple of God's spirit? It is one of the Fine Arts; I had almost said, the finest of the Fine Arts.

—Florence Nightingale

The art of nursing reaches back to when human society began. Nurses have always cared for people. No community has existed without nursing care. Nurses are everywhere: In the emergency departments awaiting casualties, in helicopters transferring critically ill trauma patients, and in hospitals where timing the respirations of 2-pound babies in neonatal units is essential. Their work is vast and comprehensive. Years and years of assessments define their knowledge base. They are the frontline caregivers and the glue to any organization, making swift decisions based on expert analysis. It doesn't matter where a trauma occurs; a nurse is always there. In the home, in the school, in psychiatric units, and in seemingly unusual places like restaurants and grocery stores. Armed with the ability to prioritize, analyze, and implement good care, nurses make the world a better place. Wherever they are working, regardless of their roles, nurses aim to help people preserve and enhance their health, well-being, and quality of life. When called upon for service, the nurse responds in the most giving of ways to make a difference.

BEING A GOOD LISTENER
by Lynn Smith (Florida, USA)

The events of September 11, 2001, have touched us all. Those of us who are nurses were frustrated more than most, because we felt so helpless in the face of such destruction. I have been a member of the federal Disaster Medical Assistance Team (DMAT) since 1998. I also have served on missions to help with the Florida forest fires and to help Houston, Texas, residents after the devastation left by tropical storm Allison. As a nurse practitioner on call for the DMAT team, I waited anxiously to hear if and when I would be deployed to New York or Washington, DC. I was eager to do something, anything, to help.

I was sent to New York on October 1, a mere 3 weeks after the "9/11" terrorist attacks. I had no idea what to expect. I knew it was a Ground Zero assignment and that we were providing assistance to the rescue and support workers there. I knew there were likely no survivors in the rubble. I did not know how I would assist with the emotional needs of the rescuers. I was worried I would not be able to keep control of my own emotions in the face of such devastation. I promised myself I would try to keep it together while I was there and worry about my own needs once I got home.

It was with great trepidation that I flew to New York. I had many questions about the safety of the scene and my role there. When we got to Ground Zero, the entire team performed a safety check of our personal gear. We also each took a minute to do what we call a "gut check," to feel the sadness of the place and decide if we felt capable of staying on. Since September 11, I had focused only on the human devastation and the stories of those who did and did not survive the collapse of the World Trade Center towers. I had packaged the event in my mind like an earthquake or natural disaster but remained focused on the victims. Seeing the destruction in person filled me with anger at the terrorists. It really hit home to me that someone had done this on purpose.

We saw many patients during our stay. We treated firefighters, police officers, telephone repair people, construction workers, and many others. Most had minor concerns, such as sprains, strains, and lacerations. Many needed their eyes washed out or remedies for the nagging coughs they had developed while working at the scene. Quite a few needed only to talk. Even weeks later, they felt compelled to tell their stories—to talk of those they had lost or of what they had seen. A number of them expressed guilt for surviving. Although our team had mental health workers available, I found the firefighters and police officers were most comfortable with nurses. I cautioned my team that we all had to be prepared to provide support, as no one could predict who would bond with whom and decide to start talking.

The patient who counted on me was a young man, an ironworker, who had come alone from Chicago to help out. The ironworkers had a very important role at Ground Zero. They were dismantling the rubble piece by piece with heavy machinery that is generally used to build things, not to demolish them. This young man came in late one afternoon and said he had a burn from the prior week he wanted examined. The burn on his outer thigh was healing well despite the fact that he had essentially ignored it. I gave him a bandage and some antibiotic ointment to cover it and some extra supplies for later, and I instructed him to keep it clean. We talked a few moments, and then he left. I wondered why he had really come. His injury seemed so small and was several days old. The next day he was back asking for another check on his wound. He asked to see me again. He had a strange look on his face, a look we had all seen a few times that week. I realized then that his minor physical need was not the reason for his visit. I checked his burn carefully. I told him he was healing well and showed him the new healthy tissue that was forming along the edges of the burn. He said, "I'm just paranoid because I am handling bodies, and I'm not used to that." The look of anguish on his face increased in intensity. We talked a long time that day. He was being asked to pull twisted metal from around some of the bodies. He had never seen a corpse prior to this job, and, at two weeks after the disaster, the bodies were in terrible shape. He told me some of the horrors he had seen, and we sat a long time quietly talking about the event. When he left he thanked me and said, "I may see you tomorrow."

He didn't come back the next day, and I never saw him again. However, I believe he was the person I most helped at Ground Zero. He did not need a great deal of physical care, but he needed a nurse to recognize his real need and respond to it. Why he chose me I will never know. Maybe it was my kind words the day before that helped him to trust me. Maybe I reminded him of someone. He probably worked there for quite awhile, as the ironworkers were there for a very long time. I only hope if he needed someone to talk to again that the DMAT nurses were still there to help him. I also hope that when he got home he was able to seek out help if he needed it. Perhaps from another nurse.

NEVER GIVING UP
by Nour O'Quinn (Florida, USA)

I am the lead, or charge, nurse on an intermediate psychiatric unit. I have a 15-year background in psychiatric nursing, and I have worked all over the world in various nursing fields. I am Lebanese. I left my country before it was torn apart in terrible fighting. I did "tent" home health with the Bedouins. I am experienced, and I thought I had seen it all. Then I met "Eddy."

I got a call from the medical unit giving report on the transfer of a young woman who was being treated medically for serious skin lesions. Her mother had brought her to the hospital because she smelled. The patient was incontinent of urine and stool, had open sores, went from mute to yelling, and was not cooperative with her treatment. Her mother tried to take her from the hospital before the transfer, hit a security guard and a nurse, and was arrested and sent to jail. "Okay," I thought, "this could be interesting."

Eddy came to the unit in a wheelchair, staring blankly into space. She appeared frightened. She wouldn't talk, walk, make eye contact, or even acknowledge that someone was there. She was about 5-feet, 4-inches, and she looked younger than her 21 years. She was underweight; had many open, weeping sores; and smelled of urine. She was positive for herpes, and had contracted hands, high white blood count, low red blood count, low hemoglobin, low protein, and low bilirubin. She was such a sad-looking girl that my heart went out to her. What had caused her to be this way?

We cleaned her, got her into bed, and discovered she did much better when only females were in the room. She cowered when men were near. "Where do I start?" I wondered. All those years of education gave me some good ideas. First, we accepted that there should be only one primary contact, and this contact should be female—me, as it turned out. Second, we needed to start building trust with her one step at a time. We also needed to maintain her hygiene, dignity, nutrition, and safety until she could start caring for herself. And lastly, we needed the whole team for input and resources.

Our plan of care focused on the essentials: We needed to get her mentally and medically stable. Eddy appeared to be actively hallucinating, and the psychiatrist started her on a new atypical anti-psychotic and added liquid nutritional supplements, antibiotics, and skin treatments to her medications. We assigned a 1:1 contact on each shift, and I took over her care. Sounded good, except she wouldn't take the medications. She would only scream when we approached her, and she wouldn't eat.

Step by slow step, things did begin to change. She began walking with assistance to the bathroom, and she let us bathe her. I set times every-day where I sat with her. "Hi, it's Nour. It is a pretty day out. I brought you a new nightgown; see what a pretty color it is." I would talk continuously or just sit and pat her hand. I kept this pattern day after day.

The social workers got in touch with a grandmother who gave us the story about Eddy. Her mother suffered from paranoid schizophrenia, and the grandmother had raised Eddy. She had graduated from high school and had plans for college, and then her mother had kidnapped her. Eddy and her mother traveled from state to state or stayed with cousins or in their car. Eddy supported them from forced prostitution work. Her mother brought her to the hospital because the sores and smell scared off the "Johns." Eddy had suffered every abuse possible, and the only retreat was into insanity. Her hallucinations were terrifying. She would yell, "Jesus Christ, help, help!" and "You're going to hell!" And then she would relapse into muteness.

My heart broke for this beautiful, young girl and the scared child inside. How could we make a difference in such a sad life? I just kept being with her. We treated her wounds, we accepted her as she was. We did our best to be her door back to normalcy, and we encouraged her independence.

As her sores healed, I brought her stylish clothes from home that my daughters had outgrown. We walked with her, talked with her, played music for her, and kept her near us. One day she looked up from her tray and said her first sentence, "Nour, I don't like this lunch. I want a hotdog." I started to cry, and you can bet she got that hotdog. She drew pictures for me in activity therapy (AT); we fixed her hair; and slowly we got to know the real Eddy. Her grandmother agreed to take her home and protect her from abusive relatives and her mother. Human Resource Services (HRS) took steps to get treatment for Eddy's mother and to make sure that Eddy would be safe. Some wounds healed, and some would always be there. The contracture in her hand from sleeping in the car improved with exercise. Finally it was time to say farewell.

The day Eddy left I felt like a mom sending her kid off to school—scared, excited, hopeful, and fearful. I knew transference and counter-transference, but I had really invested myself in Eddy, and I felt like I really did make a difference in her life. Eddy, it seemed, did too. She hugged me goodbye and said a tearful thank you. "College," she said.

BUILDING TRUST
by Iris DaCosta (Florida, USA)

This incident concerns a 49-year-old female who I shall call "Ann." She was diagnosed with paranoid schizophrenia when she had her first psychiatric admission at age 16. Since then, she has had multiple admissions. Ann was married when she was 17, but she subsequently was divorced. Ann's formal education was 8 years of school. Ann has only worked for 1 month as an adult. She receives social security insurance benefits. She displays paranoid behavior and engages in frequent physical aggression because of poor impulse control. When I first met Ann, she was living alone and was socially isolated. Ann was also depressed and withdrawn. Her only source of social support was her church, and she had stopped attending services.

Initially, I had to build rapport with her. Her social skills had deteriorated, and, combined with her paranoia, this made interactions difficult. Ann's self-esteem was poor. She never discussed herself in a positive manner. Family members reinforced this negativity, reminding her that if she worked she would lose her benefits. "I'll never be anything," Ann would say. In addition, she frequently would not take her medication.

My first goal involved teaching her about her illness and the importance of taking her medication as prescribed, as well as keeping her prescriptions filled. Her self-perception was bad; she believed that her illness was a result of her being an intrinsically bad person. I was afraid she might become involved with legal authorities because of her aggressiveness or that she might injure herself. I had to work very hard to explain her personal responsibility to herself and others and what the consequences of her behavior could be. I taught her simple and easily understandable anger-management techniques.

After she understood the importance of her medication and the reasons for controlling her anger, Ann said that she was ready to get a job. I believed that volunteer work would be a good entry into the work world. We explored possibilities, and she chose a good environment in which to begin. She decided to volunteer at a local hospital. In this way, I was available for support, and she was in a "protective" environment. Once she began volunteering, Ann also began attending church services again. At times, she would come to me for suggestions and help because the job was overwhelming to her. Simple clerical tasks such as filing were difficult for her. I had to structure situations in which she could succeed. I would role-play with her on how, for example, to accomplish a filing task she had never performed. I got index cards, put names on them, and demonstrated how to alphabetize them. In spite of my help, she lost this volunteer position.

She then withdrew and stayed at home all day. I made a home visit and was shocked to discover that she had pinned her curtains closed; in effect, she had shut the world out. Her apartment complex and her dwelling were both very dark and depressing. She acknowledged feeling depressed and had again stopped going to church. We talked, and I asked what she could see from her balcony window—the one with the curtains pinned shut. As I was talking in a soothing voice, I moved toward the window, all the while sharing with her the importance of sunlight and how people pay to visit sunny and bright tropical areas to get some of this precious sunlight. She listened and then gestured for me to unpin the curtains that had been shut so long that the pins had left rust marks on the faded cloth.

After this, she showed me around her little apartment and shared her photo album with me. I thought this indicated a level of trust that is very difficult for individuals with paranoia to experience. In addition, it suggested transference in that she might have perceived me to be someone she welcomed into her family. I felt it was critical to get Ann out of the dark environment into the light of day. She agreed, and the minute we emerged into the sunlight, her mood lifted. She became more animated. I emphasized in a brief teaching moment that this uplifting feeling she was experiencing would come again when she would go to church or engage in other out-of-home activities.

Ann began to call me often and would sometimes come to see me. Ann's disposition brightened, and her appearance improved, especially her clothing, as she was dressing in bright colors. She had begun to shop for clothing and makeup. She expressed the desire to get out of the house and interact with people. I suggested she consider working for Goodwill. She had an interview, and they accepted her and trained her for employment. Additionally, Goodwill provided classes to help her improve her academic skills in math and English.

At this time, she is awaiting job placement. She has not been in the hospital for 19 months; she is again attending church services; and she is interacting and socializing more. She has indicated over the phone with me that she is aware of the potential consequences concerning her anger-management issues. When individuals become confrontational now, Ann walks away. Throughout my work with Ann, I have continued to offer supportive therapy and acknowledgment to reinforce her gains.

RECOGNIZING THE PATIENT'S VOICE
by Meg Gambrell (North Carolina, USA)

I love being a nurse. My mother was a nurse, and I remember her coming home with stories of how she helped a patient and the impact patients had on her life. I knew that I wanted to be able to have that effect on someone someday. So I entered nursing. I had not been a nurse for very long, about 6 months, when I met the patient who made me the nurse I am today.

Sam was a 50-year-old patient who was diagnosed with Guillain-Barré syndrome (GBS). GBS is an inflammatory disorder of the peripheral nerves that is characterized by rapid onset of weakness in the lower extremities, which progresses to generalized weakness, including weakness of the muscles used for breathing. These patients are paralyzed until the inflammation subsides and muscle strength returns. This is often a lengthy process, over several months, as was the case for Sam. There is no known cause for GBS, and treatment is similar to that of a paralyzed patient until the symptoms vanish.

Sam's GBS was so severe he required a tracheostomy (a tube in the trachea) to maintain respiratory exchange. Sam had no muscle movement in his body except for weak eye blinking. He could not speak, so communication was an especially frustrating process. He kept a notepad next to him at all times. In order to facilitate communication, the nursing staff or his family would call out every letter of the alphabet. Sam would blink when you got to the letter of the word he was trying to spell. This was a very long and taxing process, for both Sam and the speller, with constant restarts and misspelled words. Just spelling the word H-E-A-D-A-C-H-E could take up to 15 minutes! At first, I was overwhelmed while caring for Sam. He and his family were anxious, and I felt helpless because frequently I could not understand what he was trying to tell me.

It wasn't until one day after Sam had developed severe pneumonia that my view of Sam began to change. Sam required suctioning every hour to keep his trachea open so he could get oxygen. Due to his paralysis, he had no cough response, and, as with everything else, suctioning was also a trying ordeal. He still could not communicate except by blinking, so I had to rely on my observations to determine if the suctioning intervention had been effective. As I advanced the suction catheter down his trachea, I noticed Sam's eyes for the first time. I had looked at his eyes numerous times for communication purposes, but I had never really looked at Sam until that moment. As I suctioned, his eyes were huge and scared. His face turned red, and his eyes looked as if they were going to bulge out of his head. He couldn't cough, he couldn't protest, he was helpless, and he was miserable. I quickly withdrew the suction catheter and stared at him. I didn't know what to say; I was so overwhelmed with emotion. Here was this man fighting for his life, fighting to breathe, and I was robbing him of oxygen. I wasn't aware of the person who I was working on; to me it was just a task that I needed to do. I was deeply ashamed of myself.

Once I regained my composure, I went through the painstaking task of asking Sam if what I had done was hurting him. Of course it was! I called in John, our respiratory therapist, and after about an hour of the "spell game" we learned that suctioning made Sam panic because it felt like "an elephant was crushing his chest," and he was oxygen hungry. My discussions with John continued, and as a result we found softer suctioning catheters that Sam tolerated better. I also became less reliant on the monitors and more aware of my patient's expressions. When I would suction Sam, I would hold my breath, and when I felt uncomfortable, I knew it was time to withdraw the catheter. Try it; it is not as long as you would think. As I began to learn more about my patient, I could tell when he needed to be suctioned—it was in his eyes. Sam just needed to look at me and I understood his need to be suctioned; our spelling game was no longer needed.

I also began to listen with my stethoscope before and after suctioning. With this method, I not only knew where the secretions were in his lungs, but I knew by listening afterward if I had adequately relieved his lungs. I also learned how far to advance the catheter in order to retrieve the secretions. Sometimes, I didn't need to listen with my stethoscope at all; I could simply put my hand on Sam's chest and feel the secretions. I knew exactly where his secretions were, how deep to advance the catheter, and how long to suction. My technique was completely different than it had been prior to Sam. We got to the point where I could just look at him and know if he was uncomfortable or in need of something. I was amazed at my new skills.

After 3 months in the intensive care unit (ICU), Sam was finally strong enough to wiggle his thumbs and speak a little. He could not move his arms or legs yet. Mouthing words was also still quite difficult because after 3 months, Sam's tongue was so atrophied that he had to practice muscle exercises—but Sam was a fighter. After an additional month, he was strong enough for a Passey-Muir valve. This speaking valve would allow Sam to communicate audibly for the first time since his illness. Together with John and Sam's wife, I heard Sam speak his first post-GBS words—he told his wife that he loved her. He then turned to me, and with slurred speech, Sam told me, "Thank you, you are my angel!"

Sam was discharged to a rehabilitation facility 7 months after his admission. During his stay, we made several other accomplishments, and we conquered many of his fears. He was an inspiration to me. A year later, Sam returned to visit our unit. He was wheelchair bound, but when he saw me, he stood up unassisted. He told me that he was making progress and the next time he came to visit we would "shag" together. I can't wait for that dance.

BELIEVING IN THE BEST OUTCOME
by Maryann Godshall (Pennsylvania, USA)

It was 6 months ago when a baby was transferred to our institution from a Philadelphia, Pennsylvania, hospital. She was one of two surviving quadruplets who were born at 24 weeks gestation to a mother who had almost died during childbirth. The patient was a baby girl I will call "Gigi." Gigi had been born in another hospital's neonatal intensive care unit (NICU), had traveled to a large inner city hospital for eye surgery, and then had traveled to Philadelphia for a tracheotomy. At 6 months of age, she was transferred to our facility to be closer to her parents, a little over an hour's drive north. We were told she was coming to our unit to die. Her condition was considered terminal. Her broncho-pulmonary dysplasia (BPD) and lung condition were the worse cases we had seen in many, many years. It was June when I first met Gigi. Her cheeks were puffed out from steroids; she existed on 70% oxygen via a ventilator with oxygen saturations in the 70s, occasionally in the 80s. To have her oxygen saturations in the 50s and 60s was not unusual. She had been on numerous types of ventilators, on nitrous oxide and many other different therapies, but all to no avail. She was evaluated for lung transplantation surgery, but she did not meet the criteria for the procedure at the evaluating hospitals. I thought this rejection would take away the last hope for her survival from her parents, but I was wrong.

Gigi had had cardiac arrest several times before coming to our hospital. What I thought would be custodial care was actually much more. Our physician tried every available therapy left, including another round of nitrous oxide. None of us thought she would live. Her condition was grave. It was her parents who never gave up. When it looked like she was going to die, they would ask, "Is there something else we could try?" Was this desperation? Or was it love?

After yet another cardiac arrest, we talked with Gigi's parents about "do not resuscitate" (DNR) orders. They agreed to sign her DNR orders, but it was a statement the father made that stuck with me throughout all the months of Gigi's care. Tearfully, he said, "I have already buried two children, I shouldn't have to bury another one." That statement stopped me cold. He was right. He shouldn't have to bury even one child, yet alone three. During this period, the family never gave up hope. It was a difficult assignment to care for Gigi, but I gladly accepted it. I didn't want to give the parents false hope, but I didn't want to take away their hope either. How could I do that? They have a right to hope and pray for a miracle.

As the 6 months went on, there were many personal, professional, and ethical concerns voiced by the staff. The bottom line to me, however, was that the plan of care for Gigi was not ours; it was ultimately the parents' decision. They had pledged to do all they could for her. I decided not only to do all I could for Gigi, but all I could for the parents. I still felt she probably would not survive, so I wanted to make their memories of Gigi as beautiful as I could. I thought even if it was the "little things," they deserved that. They deserved time to be with Gigi. They deserved a first bath picture. They deserved a picture of the two girls together. All they really wanted was for someone to care about their little girl. I know they wished someone would love Gigi as much as they did. They wanted someone to take the time to hold her, to sing to her or read to her—someone who would just take time to do the basics. I knew I could do that for them.

Gigi was the best-dressed girl in the unit. Her room was decorated for each holiday. I know it was something Gigi's mom believed she could do for her. I knew she had some guilt about celebrating the holidays with the other child at home while Gigi was still in the hospital. The parents brought in music for Gigi to listen to. Her favorites were the rock groups Journey and Pink. She had a wonderful developmental mobile over her bed. She seemed to watch and be soothed by the mobile. It wasn't until her last month with us that we found out that Gigi was profoundly deaf and blind. I had to realize the music might have been more for us, the staff, than for Gigi. But was it the music that encouraged us to provide the relaxed and non-hurried care she responded to? Or was it something else?

Even in the face of these newly discovered handicaps, the parents remained hopeful. They were clear that they would accept Gigi with whatever handicaps she had; they just wanted to take her home. It was their love for her and caring that continually motivated me. Many of the staff didn't understand why I loved caring for Gigi. I'm not quite sure myself, but there was something. Was it her spirit to live? I have never seen any child go through as many treatments, transfers, setbacks, problems, and eight cardiac arrests and still make it. I was amazed by the strength, spirit, and hope the parents displayed.

As we celebrated Gigi's 1-year birthday in the hospital, it was hard to comprehend that this child had yet to go home from the hospital. The parents called every day and came in as much as they could during the week. They took turns visiting on the weekend. Saturday was dad's day, and Sunday was mom's day. I was amazed at their unending devotion. I wondered if it was me in their situation, would I have been as devoted and have had as much faith as they did? A year! As the time progressed,

I continued to try to do those small things for the parents. They seemed little things to me, but I tried to hold her at least once a day; I tried to put her in her swing or infant seat every day; I tried to help her gain head control; I tried to do her physical and occupational therapies even when others teased me (as they thought these attempts were futile). I dressed her in a special outfit with a bow in her hair when I knew her mom or dad was coming. I listened and was supportive of her parents. I tried to be realistically honest, yet kind, when they asked the tough questions. I tried to make people see that Gigi's life, which might not be perfect in our judgment, was a life deserving of our time and respect. I tried to empathize and give the family those little things they needed when other staff members thought it was wrong. I tried to use humor to lighten up those tough times. I tried to just love this child as if it were my own. I tried to help, if even just a little. I realized that these things I did were the product of the parents' belief in their child.

After 6 months on our unit, Gigi was transferred to a rehab facility to make the transition to home. The last night she was in our unit, just a few weeks before Christmas, the mother brought us a small Christmas tree and a present. The present was a plaque with a wind chime design that said "Believe." I got the message. So many of us hadn't believed, myself included, in the beginning. The parents always believed. When a positive outcome seems far from reality, sit back and reflect on this story and try to believe.

Nurses are short on time, yet they somehow find magic moments that create the most incredible memories in their careers. Bound by paperwork and short of hands, sleep, and energy, nurses are rarely short of "caring." Their time is often spent going where no one else will go, at the bedside with frightened patients, in a high-rise with the elderly, in a home that may be unsafe. They are with patients who are on therapies that alter their senses and render them powerless. Nurses are found caring for the sick who have pain and distress. Sometimes, it is only the nurse who cares. It may seem odd, but nurses treasure these moments, live for these moments, and keep coming back for these moments.

MAKING TIME COUNT
by Connie Shepherd (Florida, USA)

"J" was a 62-year-old female who lived with her significant other and her dog. She had six adult children from a previous marriage. J was a hospice nurse and a co-worker and friend of mine.

It was December, and J, a heavy smoker, sought medical treatment for persistent, unwanted weight loss. She underwent testing and in February was diagnosed with cancer that had metastasized to the liver and adrenal glands. The doctor told J her prognosis was poor, but treatment with chemotherapy or radiation might buy her more time. Being a hospice nurse, she understood the effects that the debilitating treatment would have on her remaining life. Thus, J elected to have palliative care with hospice, and she requested that I be assigned as her primary nurse.

On my first visit, J asked if I would be okay caring for her. She said if it was going to be too hard for me she would understand. With a lump in my throat, I told her it would be much harder for me to not be the nurse caring for her. During this initial visit, we also began formulating the care plan and discussing her fears and the goals she had for the rest of her life.

J's biggest fear was having the "death rattle." J laughed as I told her that I would not allow my patients to rattle before they died. It turned out

J's concern was not for herself but for her significant other. She did not want a rattle to be his last memory of her. I reminded J that I would be able to control the rattle with medication, which greatly relieved her fear.

J had one additional fear, which was dying in pain. She knew from her hospice nursing experience that her pain would be effectively managed, but again, she needed reassurance from me that this would be the case.

J's personal goals were more challenging. Her relationship with her children had been strained since she moved to Florida 14 years prior. Even though they were grown at the time, the children felt J had abandoned them. She needed and desperately wanted to make peace with them before she died. She also wanted to put her affairs in order, such as choosing a funeral home, writing her own obituary, and planning her memorial service—if she decided to have one. Finally, she wanted to say goodbye to her sister.

J also made several demands: No hospital bed, no catheter, and she would not allow her kids to watch her die. She did not want her dying to be their last memory of her. I told J that I bet she would change her mind and want her children beside her when she died. She shook her head no and laughed at me.

As I performed my nursing assessment of J, I learned she was not sleeping well. She had no difficulty falling asleep, but she would wake up soon afterwards and realize her situation was not a dream. She had cancer and was dying. She cried, and I held her. I told her the only difference between the two of us was she knew approximately when she would die, what she was dying from, and basically how her death would occur. I, on the other hand, could be killed in a traffic accident leaving her house and would not get to accomplish the things she was going to accomplish. J hugged me and smiled. I ordered her some anxiety medication to help her sleep and to use if she needed it. J had no pain and said she had actually never felt better. We decided I would visit weekly. J's goals for the week were to get her hair done as usual and to keep living her life.

On my next visit, J told me she had spoken with her children. Together they had decided to visit in groups of two, with the first two coming the next week. We discussed what she wanted to achieve during their visits. She told me about the two children who were coming first. She shared stories about their childhoods, and she shared that she was not sure how to talk to them now. I told her she should share with them the same stories she had told me and tell them what each one meant to her. I also suggested she use the hospice social worker to mediate if she thought she needed the support. J agreed to this and seemed relieved. Our other plan was to have J take a break in the middle of the visit so she could regroup and so that the children could have some time with each other. I also told J that I would change my visit day that week and come the day the children left, because I knew saying goodbye was going to be harder than she thought. I told her to use the anxiety medication that morning, and she agreed.

J had chosen a funeral home, had contacted the hospice chaplain, was writing her obituary, and had started planning her memorial service. She was getting her affairs in order.

J had no physical complaints except that her appetite had declined. I ordered her an appetite stimulant, which I told her would not only increase her appetite but would also boost her energy level. The side effect could be a moon face, but J said to order the medication anyway.

On my next visit, J was round-faced from the medication, and she was tearful when talking about saying goodbye to the children. The visit, she said, had gone even better than she had expected. She had taken my advice and told the children stories, and she had shared her feelings with them. They left having a better understanding of why she moved and how very much she had always loved them.

The next two children would be coming in 3 weeks. She thought the appetite stimulant was a miracle drug. She was eating and felt great. J's significant other had overheard me tell her she could eat whatever she wanted, especially as much chocolate as she wished, and he had started buying her a new box of candy every week, accompanied by her favorite flowers. J was thrilled.

Three weeks went by quickly, and the next two children were arriving the next day. Again, I discussed with J the children who would be visiting. I had become her sounding board. The plan was the same: Share stories with the children, have the social worker meet with the children, and take a break. J was anxious, but ready. Again, I would visit the day the children were to leave. We now called it "my visit after."

Once again J was tearful, relieved, and happy that another visit had gone well, but she was concerned about her son. She thought he was too quiet. He was her youngest child and only son. I encouraged J to call him later for her own reassurance.

I visited the day before the last two children arrived. J was extremely anxious. I asked her why, and she said that one of the daughters to arrive the next day was the one she thought she had never bonded with—not even when she was a baby. J shared with me that this daughter and the next were only 13 months apart. The older one was only 4 months old when J became pregnant. The pregnancy had been very difficult. J had not been able to care for the older child during the entire 9 months, and their relationship had been difficult all of her life. I asked her if her daughter knew this, and she said no. I told her she needed to share this with her. J agreed.

After this visit, there were tears of joy not sadness. The visit had been very meaningful. J thought she and her daughter had found common ground. Her daughter had a better understanding of their relationship, and J felt they had bonded. Her goal was achieved.

Four months had passed since her diagnosis, and J was starting to experience weakness in her legs. I suggested a cane and got her one. J called me and said she hated it. She liked holding on to the furniture better. I laughed and told her to keep it. Around July 1, 5 months after diagnosis, J started asking, "How much longer do I have?" I told her I would turn 40 on July 18, and that she would be there for my birthday.

J still had no pain but was using a mild pain pill at night to help her sleep. Her anxiety level varied and was controlled with medication.

Two days after my birthday, J died. I went to her death. She died sitting up on the sofa with her children, her significant other, and her dog at her side. She did not rattle, did not die in pain, and did not have a catheter or a hospital bed. She had successfully died the way she set out to, with her fears avoided and her goals met. I won the bet about the children—they were at her side.

I asked her children and significant other if they wanted the hospice chaplain to attend the death. They did. The chaplain came, prayed, and sang a song J had chosen, "How Great Thou Art." At just the time he sang the lyrics "I hear the rolling thunder," it started thundering outside as if J were going out with the rolling thunder.

On my last visit with J, she told me goodbye, thanked me for caring for her, and told me she would miss me. I will always treasure my time with her.

We often talked about the gifts cancer gave her. She felt it was a gift of time—time to smell the flowers, to walk on the beach, to watch sunsets, to look at the moon, to eat whatever she wanted. It was a time to resolve family issues, time to enjoy unconditional love, and, the greatest gift of all, time to prepare for her death.

Important work is not always extraordinary. It may be a special touch, advocacy, or the little things that make a big difference. It might be just spending time with patients, talking with the families, accompanying patients to the operating room, holding a hand, sharing a story, or meeting the grandchildren; the little things go a long way. It may be as little as a handshake, a cup of coffee, or a quick game of tic-tac-toe. Despite the hectic pace in every care setting, nurses find the time and are glad they do.

CARING FOR THE ENTIRE PATIENT
by Carolina Jenson (*The Healer's Art*, p. 35)

Nurses spend a lot of time trying to help the physical body. We also need to learn the healer's art, so we can heal the body and the soul. Too often, we have preconceived notions of patients that limit our ability to care for the entire patient.

At each shift change, nurses give report about their patients' conditions to the oncoming nurses. I was receiving the usual report, and the nurse from the previous shift was determined to inform me of my patient's long history. The nurse informed me the patient had multiple visits to the emergency room (ER) the past 2 years, with various symptoms like abdominal, hip, leg, and shoulder pain; headaches; general malaise; nausea and vomiting; and decreased musculoskeletal functionality. As the nurse continued describing the patient, I thought this patient needed to have a listening ear. I would try to fulfill all her needs and listen to her questions and opinions to the best of my ability. I was going to suspend judgment for that day and serve my patient instead.

The patient awakened as I carefully poked my head into her room. She hadn't slept well, and she was in horrific and intense pain from the incision site following her exploratory abdominal surgery of the day before. I got some pain medication for her right away and then suggested ways to manage her pain for that day. We decided I would give her pain medication as often as ordered, if she felt she needed it. If that was not enough, she would let me know, and I would call the physician. Pain control was our goal, and I trusted her to know her own body. Immediately I could tell she was relieved and was able to relax.

The day progressed and I ran all over caring for my other patients. However, I took extra time to check on this woman and to enter her room to ensure that her pain was controlled. While in the room, I handed her a toothbrush with toothpaste on it, helped her brush her hair, straightened her pillow and linens, handed her a cool wash cloth to wipe her face, and got her some crackers and juice. If she could feel good about herself, then she could focus on the healing of her body. I continued to check on her frequently, and as I did, we laughed together and had deep discussions despite the fact that the actual time I was in the room was brief. Problems no one had mentioned in the report surfaced. We were able to talk about some of these problems, and she was able to think of alternative ways of dealing with the issues she was facing.

The day was extremely busy, and I was tired. At times I wanted to just take a break, sit down, and rest my weary feet. This particular day, I prioritized the patient's needs. When asked, I hurried to obtain pain medication to relieve her discomfort, as I had decided I would. Although I felt a little overwhelmed with all the things I had to do, I was able to fulfill each task and responsibility well. As I look back, I still do not know how I fit everything that needed to be done into my schedule, but I know I received strength and capacities I normally do not have.

As the day went on, we managed the woman's pain with repositioning, heat, and medications. When I looked at her chart and compared this day to the previous one, I noticed she had less pain medication on the day I cared for her. I not only cared for her medical problem, but cared for her body and her soul. I could tell she felt listened to and understood. Also, at the end of the day, she expressed gratitude for my efforts to care for her. On the opinion questionnaire patients fill out as they leave the hospital, she wrote a note and thanked me for my efforts to meet her needs.

STAYING TRUE TO THE PATIENT'S WISHES
by Francine Zabkar (Florida, USA)

"G" was a tall, pale, stoic, well-kept gentleman, looking much older than his age of 66. Piled neatly on his head were a few thin, gray strands of brittle hair, complementing his long, salt-and-pepper handlebar mustache. He had clear blue eyes, with just a hint of green, but behind those eyes I could tell was a lot of hidden pain. Not just G's physical pain, the reason he was in the intensive care unit (ICU), but there was emotional pain as well. I sensed that G had a story to tell, but I knew that I had to meet his immediate needs now.

You see, G came to me from post-anesthesia recovery, sedated and on a ventilator after having undergone an elective abdominal aortic aneurysm repair. Upon my initial assessment, I noticed that he was easily scared and agitated and experienced a lot of abdominal discomfort. I immediately reassured him that he was safe, his operation was over, and his surgery had gone well. While looking through his chart for post-operative orders, I came across his living will. I scanned it, noting in large letters he had scrawled "NO RESUSITATION!" and then beneath that he had written, "Doctor, do a good job!" That had brought a smile to my face as I realized what a grand sense of humor he had, even as he was preparing to get things in order. I'm sure that he felt very alone as he filled out the paperwork for his surgery.

Following doctor's orders, I attempted to keep him as comfortable as possible with the appropriate measures of verbal reassurance and physical comforts such as repositioning, bathing, and body massage, as well as with administering liberal doses of sedation and pain medication.

When G's pulmonologist felt the time was right to wean him from the ventilator, things went well. His arterial blood gar (ABG) results were great, and shortly after extubation he was breathing comfortably on 3 liters of oxygen via nasal cannula. But to me, something did not feel quite right. Call it "nurse's intuition," but I made a mental note to check G frequently and try to look beyond the obvious.

Since admission to my unit, G had kept his eyes closed. At first, I had attributed this to pain, fear, and just plain wanting to ignore the whole situation, something that is quite common for ICU patients after surgery. But I thought that once G was extubated, he would come around, open his eyes, speak to us, and begin to act normal. Boy, was I wrong!

After extubation, G just laid there, eyes closed, and mute. When I would call his name, or tweak his arm, he'd just grunt, "Harrumph!" Occasionally, he'd holler out, "What do you want?" Rarely would he open his eyes, halfway, not really focusing on anything, and then close them again. My heart went out to this man who seemed to be locked inside of his body.

Then, on post-operative day four during my morning assessment, I noticed a cyanotic area on the tip of G's great toe. "Oh, no!" I thought, "Could it be that he's had a cholesterol shower?" As I palpated his abdomen, I watched as he winced when I gently touched his lower-right quadrant. "Not a dead bowel," I prayed. I mentioned these findings to my co-workers. Our unit is famous for brainstorming. We like nothing better than to bounce queries and ideas off each other. Putting our heads together and utilizing the many years of experience and knowledge found in our ICU has given us many positive results for our patients. Gathering this data, I approached G's surgeon as he made rounds that morning and was prepared to bring G's climbing blood urea nitrogen (BUN) and creatinine to the physician's attention.

G had only one visitor during his entire admission. It was his cousin, H. Cousin H was more like a brother to G. They grew up together and H would sit by his cousin's bedside and talk about the good old days, never getting a reaction from G. Each day, when he arrived, he'd ask for a condition update on his cousin. I could see in his eyes that he knew it could be bad news but prayed it would be good. He hung on to each positive word I said.

"After all," he said, "G and I are buddies. We're all we have!"

It was that day, post-op day four, that Cousin H told me G's secret. When G was 35 years old, he was out for a drive with his wife and three children. After coming to a stop at a four-way crossing, looking all ways, then going ahead, a speeding car came out of nowhere and hit them broadside. His entire family was killed on impact. He was the only survivor. After that incident, G went into a deep depression. He blamed himself for the accident—if only he'd left the house 5 minutes earlier, or later, or had taken a different route, or left them at home. He had a million reasons why things could have worked out differently. No matter how hard H tried to reason with him, G always felt the same guilt.

During daily visiting hours, H religiously shaved G. He told me that G was a very meticulous man and would never go one day without shaving. I would hold the breathing tube out of the way and move it so that H could diligently get to each crevice in G's face. Because he himself was elderly, it took him a long time to do the job, but even at my busiest, I made time to assist him, knowing this was the only way he knew to show his love.

G never flinched as Cousin H lathered him and glided the razor over his face, without ever nicking him. After he was done, Cousin H would say goodbye and come back the next day and repeat the same scenario. I could tell that this ritual was therapeutic for both of these old-timers.

Then, the inevitable happened. On post-operative day five, all of G's doctors had a conference. He did indeed have a dead bowel, needed surgery and dialysis, and would probably have to have a below-the-knee amputation of his leg.

When I heard that, I stepped up to the plate as my patient's advocate. Poor G! He couldn't, or wouldn't, speak for himself! I brought out his living will. Showing it to these doctors, I explained that he requested "no heroics," how he'd been depressed all his life about the accident that happened more than 35 years ago, and how he'd have no problem going to be with his dear family!

The doctors stopped talking, listened to what I had to say, and then proceeded to discuss their plan for taking G to the OR. "The best we can do is dialyze him, open him up, do an e-lap and colostomy, cut the leg off, and put him in a nursing home for the rest of his life. Send him to the OR in an hour. Oh, and call Cousin H for permission."

"No" I said, "YOU call Cousin H." And I turned on my heels and left the room. I went directly to G's bedside and took his hand in mine.

"I'm so sorry, G." I said. "Your living will means nothing, it's just a piece of paper! I tried to fight for you, but now all I can do is pray that you will be all right!" With that, I may have imagined it, but I swear, I felt G squeeze my hand.

Cousin H did indeed give permission for the surgeries. He wanted G to live, at all costs, in any condition. After all, G was all that H had in life! I had to realize that I was just an outsider, trying to understand where he was coming from.

That afternoon, G came back to me from the OR, on a ventilator again. His blood pressure was 70/40 and he was in supra ventricular tachycardia (SVT). He had no urine output, his temperature was 94.2, and he was ashen. They had done their surgery, and I believed they had "done him in."

To my amazement, G made it through that surgery. In 4 days, the colostomy was functioning well, and he began to come around. His vital signs had also stabilized. Now our concern was weaning him from the ventilator again. We had hoped that he would do well. Monitoring his oxygen saturation levels closely, we suctioned him, provided nebulizer treatments, and assisted his respiratory efforts in every way possible. But he eventually tired, and his ABGs were indicative of the need for re-intubation.

One week later, after multiple weaning attempts, an ear, nose, and throat (ENT) specialist was consulted, and I sent G off for a tracheostomy. I cringed. "Here we go again." I just kept thinking about G's living will. It just seemed so redundant to mutilate the body of someone whose desire was "no heroics." Cousin H was now beginning to feel guilty and had reservations about signing permission forms, but I found myself actually encouraging him to do so. After all, NOW was not the time for him to go on a guilt trip! We'd already gotten this far!

G had his tracheostomy the next day, and he tolerated it well. He was dialyzed every other day. Things started to look better. He was on day 16 of his hospitalization when he began to spike a temperature ... 101.3 ... 102.2 ... 102.9 ... 103.1. Now he was becoming septic. Another setback!

Finally, the infectious disease specialist was consulted. "Man, I was so surprised to see G on my list," he said to me. "I just saw him in my office last month for a UTI (urinary tract infection). What a super guy! Great sense of humor … reminded me of the comedian Bob Hope. On each office visit, he'd wear a funny, different hat. I really hate seeing him like this. He's a fighter, to say the least. I'm sure that's why he's made it this far! I'm going to do my best to help him get over this infection and move on. G loves life too much to give up!"

When I heard this doctor's words, I thought to myself, "Loves life to much to give up …" Maybe it was I who was giving up all this time! Maybe, by trying to be what I thought was G's advocate, I was misinterpreting what I thought his quality of life ought to be!

Then I closed my eyes and pictured G in a nursing home, in a wheelchair, with an ostomy, and with a leg without a foot. But he was wheeling around, wearing a funny hat, doing Bob Hope impersonations, telling funny stories, and making others laugh. It was then that I realized that maybe my idea of "quality of life" and my patient's idea might be very different. From now on I will try to look at my patients' situation from their viewpoint and not let my values get in the way.

I thought this was the end of my story and my lesson learned. Four months later, I was reading the obituaries, as so many nurses do, and there it was … I did a double-take. After all the work we did, all that praying, G died anyway!

The obituary was a short memoir of how G, a widower and war veteran, had moved to Florida 20 years ago with his cousin H and how they had built and designed their home. The memorial service for G was that night.

I decided right then and there to do something I had not done in many years. I had to say goodbye to G just one more time. I planned to sneak in at the end of the service, mix with the crowd, and leave without being noticed. I wanted to get lost among the others—just get in and get out. I was afraid that if my eyes met with H's, I'd lose it, and after all, that would not be very professional.

As I pulled my car up to the funeral home, I saw only the hearse; a shiny, black limo; and an older, simple, tan compact car with handicap plates. I checked the newspaper again to be sure that I had the right location, date, and time. Yes, this was the place. I entered through the heavy, mahogany doors.

After my eyes adjusted to the darkness, I spotted a sign to the right, near an entrance to a small room, with G's name on it. I peeked in and saw no one but H sitting in the front pew, all alone, staring at the closed casket, his back to me. Upon the casket was a black-and-white photo of a very dashing, debonair, laughing G with his handlebar mustache with his shy, pretty wife, surrounded by their three mischievous-looking young boys sitting on a blanket in a park having a picnic.

Near the picture were four hats, all lined up in a row. The first one was from the Chicago railroad where G had worked, the next was a New York Jets cap, G's favorite football team. Next was a black "Old Fart's Club" cap, and lastly was his worn and tattered beret from the U.S. Army.

I walked into the softly lit room and approached H, laying my hand on his shoulder. He turned his head and looked up to me. He didn't need to speak. I could read the sadness in his tearful eyes. I leaned down, and we hugged for what seemed like an hour, but it was only moments. I said I was sorry, he said he was too. Then I sat down beside him. We held hands and stared at the casket, silently, until the funeral director told us it was time to leave. H gathered up G's picture and hats and walked me out to my car. As I opened my car door, he handed me G's New York Jets cap. "Here," H said, "remember our buddy." I took the hat reverently, laid it on the seat next to me, and drove home. It was then that I realized that nursing takes place in more areas than just a hospital ... it could be in a funeral home, a parking lot, a car, and most of all ... in one's heart!

Assessing, Communicating, and Persevering
by Penny Kochanowski (Florida, USA)

He was only 19, at the prime of his young adulthood, yet still a child to his parents. Suddenly, a motor vehicle crash changed everything. "T" sustained multiple injuries. His Glasgow Coma Scale was three on arrival to the unit. He was not wearing a seat belt at the time of the crash. T was assigned to my care after emergency treatment.

I started the day after receiving report as I usually do. I reviewed the chart and medication record, and then I went to the room to see T. After introducing myself and assessing him, I left the bedside. I looked back at him one more time as I was leaving the room. I noted that he kept his head turned to the right. I reviewed the chart again, searching for any documentation regarding this finding; there was nothing.

I consulted with another nurse who had cared for this patient. She said his neck was slightly turned to the right but not as much as it was now. The spine films showed no evidence of acute fracture or subluxation—even though he had a surgical repair of the mandibles. The patient's father said that T's neck had been turned to the right for a few days. I told the charge nurse of this abnormal finding and summoned the doctor. He examined the patient but was not impressed.

I continued to monitor him and repeatedly contacted the doctors on service, each time stressing the fact that even when the patient was turned to the left, he kept his head to the right. I also managed to tell them that this was not normal. Finally, in the early evening, deep concern overcame me. I couldn't go off duty with a clear conscience knowing my patient could be in danger.

I consulted a doctor on the unit from another service. The request was simple: Please come to my patient's room and give me your opinion. After I explained the situation, he was very accommodating and accompanied me to the bedside. Dr. S required I call his primary doctor, which I did immediately. The order given by the primary doctor was to "place an aspen collar on the patient." I paged the ortho tech to assist with this order.

When the ortho tech arrived and saw the patient's head rotation, he refused to apply the aspen collar. Dr. S, too, was not interested in rotating this young man's neck. Dr. S ordered a STAT neurosurgery consult, and they placed the collar on the patient.

The next day the client was diagnosed with "torticollis"—a spasmodic condition of the neck. Things still did not seem exactly right, and with further questioning the chief neurosurgeon reviewed the films and found the young man to have a congenital defect of his spine. The condition is known as "Os Odontoidium." The patient was emergently supplied with Garner-Wells tongs in his skull and placed on a rotorest bed to stabilize his neck. He then went for a bone fusion. Dr. S informed me that this congenital anomaly would have eventually weakened, causing a spontaneous fracture that would have rendered this young man paralyzed from the neck down. The two doctors came to me and thanked me. One said, "You saved all of us. I told all of my students to listen to you; they could learn from you. Good call; good job."

Every day we do our assessments, give our medications, establish and administer IVs, and assist with the many facets of patient care. We are continually required to communicate with everyone we come in contact with, in a personal manner. The demand for highly advanced skill levels is imperative to meet the physical aspects of care. The bottom line, however, is to make a difference every day in some way. We need to go back to the essential, basic skills we first learned in nursing—assessment, communication, and perseverance—because they really make the difference. The young man in this story is still walking because of these basics.

TAKING TIME TO CARE
by Jonna Barker (Illinois, USA)

The crying patient was a lady whom I had cared for during my education. She was suffering from dementia. I walked into the room and asked her what was wrong. She cried more, saying she felt so confused and just "not herself."

In frustration, with tears in her eyes, she told me she could not find her grandson's phone number. We looked all over her room and at the nurses' station before we finally found it. I helped her dial the number and then I began to gather my things and walk out of the room. After all, I had been nice and helpful already, and I had a lot of other things to do.

As I approached the door, I heard her hang up the phone. I thought, "I really hope her grandson will visit, especially since she didn't get to speak with him. She really needs someone to talk to." As this thought crossed my mind, I froze. Who was I? What was my role? I turned around, leaving my worries about myself at the door. I walked back in and sat beside this wonderful person. As I did so, her eyes lit up, and we began talking. She told me about her past; she recalled her age and the year she was born—information she could not provide during the previous week. Her depression and gloom transformed into happiness. She talked of her younger years, and we found that we had much in common. We had a very meaningful, heartfelt discussion. As I prepared to leave, she told me how much she loved her family and that she felt like I was part of her family. She was peaceful and calm.

As I left her room, my heart was filled with joy from this simple act of service. I learned an important lesson that day. My life was blessed as I took the time to go beyond being "nice" and truly care for this patient. Suddenly my worries were forgotten and my burdens were lifted. I learned that nursing is more than clinical skills or fulfilling assignments.

REFLECTIONS FROM A NEW NURSE
by Vanessa Cox (Queensland, Australia)

There is one patient and his family that will leave a special imprint in my memory and my heart. He was an elderly gentleman admitted with a bladder neoplasm. During his admission, he underwent a cholecystectomy, a right iliac artery aneurysm repair, and an evacuation of a hematoma. This man was in severe pain, and during morning report it was communicated that the nurses had only to lift the blankets from his body and he would scream in pain and yell verbal abuses. The shift report indicated he was uncooperative with assessments, interventional measures, medications, and diet, and it also described his family as being somewhat difficult. As I prefer to make my own appraisal of people, I did not alter my behavior based upon the latter remarks. Luckily, my instincts and outlook proved advantageous for this patient and his family.

I was wary of this patient at first as I am very conscious of inflicting pain, and his pain levels were disturbing to me. As I entered his room, the first thing I did was try to talk to him. He was unresponsive to me immediately, and his verbal and non-verbal behaviors indicated severe pain. He kept his eyes closed and frequently winced with pain, his face showing a constant grimace. Before I began assessing him, he communicated with me a little more but kept his eyes closed. By the end of my assessment, I found that he had varied areas of skin breakdown that were not mentioned in report. I continued to communicate with him during the time I was in his room, and by the time I finished my assessment, he had opened his eyes and was talking directly with me. The only trouble I had was that he could not roll onto his side independently as he was in so much pain.

The magnitude of his pain was very alarming to me. I discussed this with my preceptor, and she said that a pain management consultant had already assessed him and he was too uncooperative to allow for any real intervention. My preceptor organized another consultation later that afternoon. This made me feel somewhat better. I spent a lot of time with this patient on my first day. Sometimes I didn't say anything, but I believed he liked me being there and was comforted by the knowledge that he was not alone. Sometimes we had short conversations, and it felt rewarding that I had progressed this far with a patient who was considered uncooperative and abusive.

The next day he remembered me and called me by my name. This seemed like considerable progress from the day before. The new analgesia had obviously started its effect. He was much more cooperative with me and rolled independently. He still had considerable pain; however, he indicated that he wanted to help me by doing what he could for me. He even smiled at me, and I felt like giving him a hug and telling him how proud I was of him. His wife came in this day, and I introduced myself to her. She was very sweet. She was genuinely concerned for the welfare of her husband, and she exhibited a need for support and hope. She was understandably very distressed about her husband's condition.

At one point, she felt so hopeless that she burst into tears and ran from his room. I followed her out and offered support. After a hug, a cup of coffee, and supportive conversation, she felt able to go back into her husband's room and find the strength to finish her visit. During my conversation with her, I identified a number of issues. She had a need for spiritual support as well as intellectual and psychological support. With her needs obvious to me, I was bothered by the description of the family as being difficult. Clearly, this woman was in some distress. My preceptor and I arranged for pastoral care for this patient and his wife, for which they were very grateful. We also contacted the physician to arrange for a meeting with the patient's wife so that she could receive information about her husband's condition and satisfy her intellectual needs. With the focus on these two needs directly, I felt that the psychological needs would be consequently satisfied.

I cared for this patient daily for nearly 2 weeks. My relationship grew with him and his wife. He even asked me to call him by his nickname, which was an honor, and he told me stories about his time in the war and in the army in general. He spoke of all the places he had traveled and how proud he was of his family. We even shared jokes, and it was so rewarding to come so far with this patient on both a physical—his outcomes were improving—and psychological level. His pain was still a major issue; however, he and I had developed a relationship that enabled us to complete assessments and interventions with minimal pain infliction. To see him smile when I came into the room was such a wonderful experience.

Even when I was nursing in different units, I went to his room during my lunch break just to say "hello" to him and his wife, and they enjoyed my presence, if only for a few minutes. It was obvious to me that when the needs of the patient and his wife were addressed, there was a complete change in his and his family's demeanors.

As I reflect back on this patient, there are a number of things that I learned. The most important lesson for me is the value of providing truly holistic care. My feelings are that the patient is more than just one entity. There exists a myriad of factors and synergy that create the person. My approach is to look beyond the medical model of care and see the real person, not just the patient, in order to individualize care to meet his or her needs, as well as the needs of the family members. I believe that the biggest learning experience I had with this patient is to follow my instincts. I learned the value of making my own appraisal of people and to never be swayed by the opinions of others who may not have had the time, or taken the time, to really get to know the patient. This is the part of nursing I love and which ignites a passion within me. It is my hope that this passion will continue to grow and serve me and my patients well for as long as I have the privilege of providing nursing care.

TAKING A RISK
by Susan Scholtz (Pennsylvania, USA)

Glancing over the list of potential patient assignments for my nursing students, my attention focused on a complex case. An elderly woman, diagnosed with advanced stage cancer, had countless treatments ordered. I envisioned many opportunities for my nursing students to provide quality nursing care while building a repertoire of skills. What I failed to realize was the impact this patient and her family would have on me, both professionally and personally.

I recall entering her room and going through the standard introductions. My initial impression of Mary was that the disease had taken its toll on her. She was pale and fragile, yet a smile illuminated her face. Immediately, a tall, robust man leaped from a chair next to her bed. Self-assuredly, he approached me and directed my attention to a newspaper clipping hanging from her television. He said forcefully, "This is my Mary. She helped create and dedicate this shrine to St. Anne. Our faith has brought us through difficult times in the past, and it will get us through this." Once these words were spoken, he retreated to his chair. The remainder of the day's events were blurred; however, I felt a connection to this family.

Over the next few weeks, Mary's condition worsened, and her husband began to reach out to me. He spoke with pride about his Italian heritage and his love for his family. He shared recipes for favorite Italian dishes and listened to my family stories attentively. His son and daughter also joined in these conversations. Each day I learned something special about his beloved Mary. Each reflection he shared about Mary's life helped me to see her in yet another dimension. Although I never knew her before she became terminally ill, he created an image of her that I will always remember. Together we planned strategies to help Mary live her final days comfortably.

One day, "S," Mary's husband, pulled a prescription pill bottle from his shirt. He handed it to me tentatively and said apologetically, "I am supposed to take these pills for my blood pressure, but I can't seem to remember to take them." I sat down with him and talked to him about the importance of taking his medication. I stressed how important it was for him to take care of his health so he in turn could be there for his wife. In addition to his wife's daily assessments, I would also measure his blood pressure. Although he assured me he had taken his medications, intuitively I knew he had not.

I will never forget the morning I entered Mary's room and saw the chair next to her bed empty. I continued to make rounds but made a mental note to return. Later in the day, I saw Mary's physician emerge from her room, and I asked if he knew where her husband was. He whispered, "He is a patient in the intensive care unit." I felt my heart sink and found myself heading to the intensive care unit (ICU). As I entered the ICU, my eyes were drawn to the corner room. Beneath countless tubes and lines was a man I could barely recognize. The robust man whose trademark was a plaid shirt and a belt with a huge buckle now seemed frail in his patient gown. As I looked toward him, he glanced at me, closed his eyes tightly, shook his head slowly, and turned away from me. I felt the tears well up in my eyes, and the composure I should have maintained as a nurse escaped me. Had I allowed myself to become too close?

Over the next few weeks, I continued to assign my students to care for Mary. Although S was too weak to visit his wife, I felt connected to him through his family. Apparently the connection was mutual. One morning the phone rang, and I immediately recognized the voice. Apparently S had a reaction to a dye, and his kidneys had stopped functioning. Tentatively he asked, "Can you come and talk with me?" Hesitantly, I approached him and found myself sitting in the chair next to his bed much in the same manner he had done with Mary. We talked about his fears and hopes for himself and shared the richness of his and Mary's life together. His faith in God was strong, and we vacillated between laughter and tears. This dialogue was to be the last one we would share. Just as this couple had been together in life, they were soon to be reunited in death.

In reflection, I realize my experience with this family had enabled me to grow professionally and personally. I also realize each time I reach out and embrace a family there is tremendous risk for inner pain;

yet the richness gleaned from immersing oneself in a nurse-patient relationship can never be replicated. Although our encounter happened over a decade ago, the feelings and commitment to the family come flooding back to me as I pay tribute to them in this story.

These stories are real; they are about the lives of nurses who truly make a difference. They are part of the nurse-life journey. You have read how nurses have given many intangible resources—reaching out to families, being an advocate, taking time, prioritizing care needs, and providing comfort measures. In the stories, you can feel the remembrance of the past and the efforts made to make life better for someone—patient, family, or both. The stories are reminders of the impact of key life experiences. This freedom to discover and share feelings they didn't even know they had has assisted many nurses in understanding the complexities and ambiguities of caring. The stories have closed the grieving.

The narratives in this chapter set a tone for future ones. Many of the themes will be expanded upon—caring, spirituality, courage, and comfort, to name but a few. As you progress through the remaining chapters, feel the wisdom of the nurse, appreciate the particular event in time, and listen with your heart.

REFERENCES

Brigham Young University College of Nursing. (2002). *The Healer's Art.* Provo, UT.

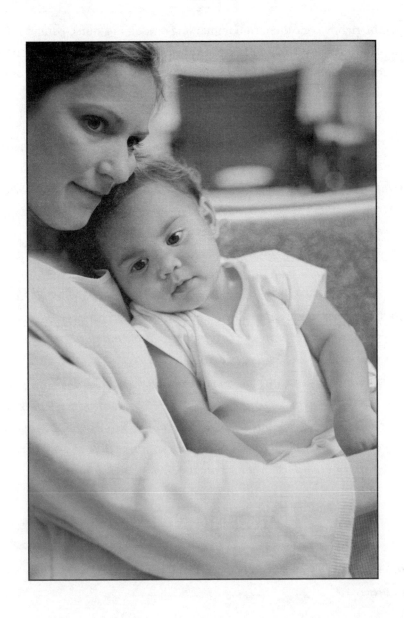

CHAPTER 2

Caring: The Essence of Nursing

Too often we underestimate the power of a touch, a smile, a kind word, a listening ear, an honest compliment, or the smallest act of caring, all of which have the potential to turn a life around.

—*Leo Buscaglia*

Caring is the core of nursing. It is an instinctual, natural part of the work of a nurse. Empathic caring—feeling the pain of another and trying to implement strategies to improve the health state—is the nurse's challenge. The best nurses create the time to care: to ask the hard, steadfast questions about the patient to improve the plan of care and investigate beyond the norm.

Caring is difficult to define. To enter a caring partnership, one has to be attentive, concerned, and knowledgeable. No one can make another care; it has to be a free offering of oneself. No one can teach the true sentiment of caring; it is a gift—a talent, not a standard. The caring nurse must feel the desire to care, rather than be told to care.

Nurses develop authentic relationships and learn how to behave professionally and communicate effectively. Over many years, they study key assessments and pathology and focus on the process and implementation of care. They gain knowledge of how best to document and evaluate care. Numerous hours are focused on therapeutic relationships and what is called the affective domain: determining care, valuing caring, and attending to caring (Krathwohl, Bloom & Masia, 1964).

Scotto (2003) challenges us to go beyond the traditional definition of caring in her writings on "A New View of Caring." This involves developing an awareness of the intellectual, psychological, spiritual, and physical integrity a nurse brings to the caring relationship. The intellectual aspect of caring is the knowledge the nurse brings to each patient. The psychological aspect of caring includes knowing how human experiences shape life. Spiritually, nurses are in varied settings supporting patients' efforts to reach their own goals. Finally, the physical part of nursing involves using all senses to deliver care.

Contemporary nurses are indeed practicing "a new view of caring." In fact, their caring relationships convey intense meaning for both themselves and the patient. Nurses of today are conscious of body, mind, and soul connections. They are dedicated to caring built on scientific knowledge. Their interactions create pride and commitment. But incredibly and consistently, their connections with patients involve empathy, warmth, trust, courtesy, and a simple but respectful honesty.

CARING BY HELPING EACH OTHER HEAL
by Maryann Godshall (Pennsylvania, USA)

In more than 100 years of professioal nursing, there is one aspect that has not changed, and that is caring. Caring is the heart of nursing. In no other specialty of nursing is caring more important than in the care provided to infants and children. Parents place their trust in the pediatric nurse's hands to care for the most cherished people in their lives—their children.

There are many areas of nursing on which to focus one's career, but one that I feel is most challenging is caring for children. I'm not talking about the technical aspects, but rather about the emotional part. It is especially challenging when dealing with children and families facing death. I've come to respect the devotion of many of my coworkers in pediatrics. In adult nursing, death is easier to deal with because most patients have already lived a good life. In pediatrics, children's lives have just begun. When death occurs, it's difficult to find any reason or rationalization for its occurrence.

When I entered nursing, I was excited and energized to "change the world." What I didn't know was how nursing was going to change me. Nursing has taught me valuable lessons, and when I reflect on these experiences, I realize the profound impact of my chosen path. What follows is the story of an experience that changed my life forever. It has made me look at nursing differently. It has made me not only a better nurse, but also a better person.

One slow Friday evening in June, while working in the pediatrics unit, we got a call from the emergency room (ER) that a pediatric code was coming. As was protocol at that time, a pediatric nurse was supposed to respond. Another nurse and I went down and took our nursing technical assistant, who was a nursing student, along for the experience. I had been back from maternity leave for about 5 months. I had been working in pediatrics for almost 2 years and felt pretty comfortable with my skills. We went to the pediatric room and got ready. We had an entire team—respiratory, anesthesia, neonatologist, pediatrician, and nurses from the ER and the pediatric unit. I was sure this was going to go smoothly. I was most comforted by the fact that I had just completed the Pediatric Advanced Life Support (PALS) class 2 months before. Everything was fresh in my mind.

The patient was an 8-month-old baby diagnosed with sudden infant death syndrome (SIDS). I was trying to put out of my mind that I had an 8-month-old at home. The ambulance arrived and to my surprise, my PALS instructor was with the ambulance crew. I had no doubt this event would have a positive outcome.

I was so very wrong. No one in the room could get a line in. We had two of the best pediatricians running the code. We did everything possible, but there was no response. Despite a lengthy resuscitation effort, the baby died.

The parents were outside and wanted to see her. The grandparents were visiting from overseas and were spending their first night with their granddaughter. The grandmother had found the baby motionless in the crib. I tried to prepare the little girl as best I could, and then I left the room. I couldn't make eye contact with the family as I heard them crying. I felt like such a failure. I cringed as I heard them openly weeping at her bedside. I had to go, but I needed to know her name. The ER staff pointed me to her Addressograph. I stamped it on a card and left.

When I reached the pediatric unit, the entire pediatric staff was in tears, especially the nursing student we took along for "the experience." I felt responsible for her as well. "What had we done?" I thought, "It wasn't supposed to work out this way." I looked at the piece of paper I had stamped and saw the little girl was 8 months old, the same age as my daughter. Their birthdays were 3 days apart. I held it together as best I could and went home.

That night, I went to my daughter's crib, picked her up, and released my emotions. I could only imagine how the other mother was feeling. I felt so lucky my world was still safe and sound. In the following days, feelings of guilt overcame me. Why had this mother lost her daughter, and I still had mine? I was grateful, of course, that it didn't happen to me, but I couldn't understand why it had happened at all. We know life is unfair, but why this child? Is there ever an answer? I felt a strong sense of the pain this mother must be feeling. The mental picture of that little girl, motionless on the litter, was haunting. I couldn't erase it from my mind. I felt the need to contact this mother with a simple card to express my sympathy. I shared with her that I, too, had an 8-month-old daughter and that I couldn't imagine her pain. I felt better after I sent the card.

About a week after that awful night, when I got to work, there was a message from this mother. She left her phone number. What did she want? What would I say? What had I done? I didn't feel strong enough to talk to her. The following Monday, after I put my daughter down for a nap, I got up the courage to call her. She wanted to know one thing: Did her Chelsey ever have a heartbeat? I wondered why she wanted to know that. I told her the ambulance crew thought they had a heartbeat in the ambulance at one point, but she never had one in the ER. I again expressed my condolences and said I would have liked to have seen a picture of her little girl prior to that night. She looked so beautiful with her curly blond hair. I hung up believing I would not speak to this mother again.

A few months passed, during which I was trying to deal with and forget that Friday night. Then one day I went to work, and there was a letter from this mother. I opened it and found a thank-you note for what I had done. "Thanking me," I thought, "For what? I hadn't saved her daughter." There were also two pictures of Chelsey sitting on the sofa playing patty-cake. You can imagine my reaction as I ran to the locker room.

A year later on the anniversary of that horrible night, I sent this mother a single pink rose and a brief note to let her know I had not forgotten about Chelsey. I thought the 1-year anniversary of that night would be awful for this mother. I wanted her to know I remembered Chelsey, even though her life was so short. The mother sent me a card back, thanking me for remembering. She told me she was pregnant and that she knew it was a girl. She and her husband planned to give the baby the middle name of Chelsey. I thought, "How beautiful." She sounded so strong in the note. I wondered if I would have been that strong had this happened to me. It was at this point that I was finally able to move on and let go of this incident. I realized this mother was accepting the tragic loss, and so should I.

I don't enjoy the excitement of a code situation, but if it arises, I deal with it. I try to keep communication lines open with the parents at all times. Anyone can be trained to handle the technical aspects of nursing. It's the psychosocial aspect of care that is the essence of who we are. It is still very hard for me to deal with children who are very ill and are the same age as my children. But I have found that if I look at these children and think about how I would want my child treated in that situation, I am able to effectively do my job. It helps me provide the empathy and support that only a nurse and a mother can understand.

I have never heard from this mother again, but that's OK. We helped each other heal through one of life's most awful experiences.

Caring requires inventive thinking. Patients and their families are devastated by chronic illnesses, hospitalization, and the loss of power. They just don't know what to do. Many develop emotional problems such as depression. This reality makes caring tough to deal with. However, paying attention to a patient's social and emotional life patterns is imperative. Nurses understand that merely starting the caring process requires listening to the patient and being non-judgmental. The bonds of trust do not occur overnight, but instead are nurtured day in and day out by nurses who take the time to care. Slowly and oh-so-carefully, a plan of care was developed in the following stories that illustrates the importance of understanding one's past. This understanding of the past—the history—leads to genuinely effective care of others in the future.

CARING BY REMOVING POWER STRUGGLES
by D'Ann Van Lente (Florida, USA)

Mr. Jones was admitted through the emergency room (ER) with congestive heart failure and renal failure related to anorexia. His wife was at his side as he was rolled by me on a gurney, and I could barely see him hidden under the covers and a nonrebreather facemask. As I lifted the covers to assist him to the bed, I found an extremely emaciated older man the color of paste, with multiple contractures. I silently asked a thousand questions as I watched every rib move each time he gasped for air. (What took him this long to get to the hospital? Why didn't his wife bring him in sooner? Why didn't she do something about his weight loss before this?) Those were the wrong questions at that time. Instead, I needed to focus on assessing his condition.

Mr. Jones was cold as I touched his hands and looked into his sunken eyes. I discovered he was refusing to eat and drink, saying he wasn't hungry and felt too weak to eat. His wife tried to cajole him into eating. She was approximately 20 years younger and ran the family business. She was impatient and couldn't understand why "he wouldn't mind." I told her I needed to assess him and begin the infusion of the first of three units of blood. I suggested she take a break and get something to eat.

I needed time to assess him. Every joint was contracted until he was in a tight ball, and he had pressure sores on all major bony prominences. I couldn't straighten his arms in order to assess his heart and lungs. I felt like I was having a wrestling match just to do my assessment. (How did this man get so contracted? Didn't this woman ever do range-of-motion exercises with her husband? What happened to home health or physical therapy?)

I tried to figure out what brought this man to this point. I pored over his medical history, looking for details that would answer my questions; I found few. He had been married 10 years, but became ill 3 years ago with weight loss and hypertension. At that time, he turned the business over to his wife. Before that point, he was active and in good health. (Could she be doing something to cause this?) The only two things in life he loved were his business and baseball. He had given up both. Now he was angry and bitter, yelling at anyone who showed kindness, and he was dying. He didn't want food, water, or units of blood.

He finally agreed to the blood transfusions. He was already in congestive heart failure, wheezing and laboring with every breath. Although he was extremely anemic, adding fluid quickly could send him into crisis. As I monitored his vital signs, I asked him about baseball and his eyes lifted. It was his one true love. He had been a pitcher. I knew then that baseball was going to be the basis for my teaching, my learning, and the path to understanding him. Baseball was going to be the way I could encourage him toward health. So every time I came into the room, I asked him another question about baseball or asked him to tell me something about a game he played. As the days passed, he looked better, his congestive heart failure was controlled, and he began to eat.

All of these changes stopped when the doctors told him their goal was to place a feeding tube in his stomach and begin kidney dialysis. When I entered his room, he was covered with blankets. His IV had been pulled out, and he was acting angry and fearful. He told me to leave him alone. I said I would give him time and would be back in a few minutes to check his vital signs. He was still acting angry when I came back. I sat quietly next to his bed and asked him what happened when a pitcher got older and his arm started to give out. He said either the coach gave him less playing time, making his arm weaker, until the pitcher realized he was too old and should give up, or the coach constantly pushed the pitcher until injuries occurred, effectively ending his career. I then asked him which kind of pitcher he had been. He said he used his arm less, got weaker, and then gave up. I thanked him for sharing and quietly checked his vital signs and restarted his IV. I didn't ask him about dialysis or tube feeding. I hoped he could see a correlation between the result of his not exercising his pitching arm and the likely result of his refusing to eat, drink, and move. In fact, the more his wife and others tried to make him eat, the more he refused.

After leaving his room, I asked his wife if we could talk to develop a plan for his care. As I sat with her, she appeared powerful. Her erect posture and broad shoulders implied confidence. I asked her about their relationship during the last 10 years and how she managed with his being sick for the last 3. She said that after he gave the business to her so he could do other things, he became more easily tired. She tried to tell him what to do for his health, but "he just wouldn't listen!" He stopped going out and stayed in bed while she was at work and after she got home. He said he wasn't hungry for dinner, and she would find breakfast and lunch thrown away. Everything she tried failed. She encouraged, begged, and argued—all without success. Now she was afraid he was going to die. She no longer appeared powerful or confident.

We discussed the paradox of power. She appeared powerful but had no power. He appeared frail and helpless but held all the power. As long as food was part of a power struggle, he would win. We needed to create the impression that his eating or not eating would not matter, and food would not be an issue. We spoke to the doctor to get his consent for the plan.

He didn't receive his dinner tray that evening. When he told me he didn't receive a tray, I reminded him that he continually said he wasn't hungry, didn't want to eat, and didn't even want to see food. I then explained I gave his tray to another patient. I told him to let me know if he became hungry. He looked confused and frustrated. Neither of us offered him food. There was no longer a power struggle. His wife said she was going to get something for dinner and would return. When she returned, she didn't bring him food but instead did paperwork. Food was not discussed again that evening. Subsequent meals were brought in the room, but no one attempted to persuade him to eat or offered to feed him. Food became a "non-issue." But I still asked him to tell me his baseball stories.

By the second day without food, his arms and hands, covered with bandages, were shades of purple from the multiple IV restarts due to collapsed veins. He finally agreed to a central line placement for the vital infusion of IV fluids. As I entered the room at the beginning of the shift, he asked for something to eat. If I had made a big deal about his eating now, he wouldn't have eaten when I brought him food. So without changing my expression, I asked what he would like to eat. He told me, and I called the cafeteria with the order. Then I called his wife. I was really excited that he wanted to eat, and I warned her to be nonchalant about his eating when she came to visit. Food needed to stay a non-issue.

Although he was now eating, his nutritional status was extremely poor. He needed tube feedings, and he wasn't understanding the correlation between his pitching career and his life. (Did he want to die, or was that something he thought was expected of him?) I again brought up the topic of pitchers leaving baseball when his wife came in that evening. I asked him if he thought it was fair that coaches pushed pitchers out of the game, and he said no. I asked him to explain how and when he would have preferred to leave baseball. He told me he wanted to leave when he was strong and healthy, "nothing too weak or broken." His wife watched me carefully. I was quiet for a minute while I said a quick prayer and took a deep breath. Then I asked, "Isn't that how you would like to die also?" When he looked up, all color left his slightly pale, pink face, and he just stared at me. "I don't think the coach meant to generalize ending your life like he taught you to end your baseball career," I added.

As he began describing the time when he left baseball, he began to cry. The coach had decided it was time for a new pitcher. Mr. Jones had thought he was getting ready for the major leagues. He was pulled from the lineup and used infrequently. After feeling embarrassed and unwanted, he resigned. He felt the same way after he got married and his wife began taking over responsibilities at work. He gave her the company and resigned from life. He didn't think he was needed. At this point, I knew they needed privacy to talk.

Later, when the call light was turned on, I entered the room. They decided he would have tube feedings and continue to eat as much as he could. He was still very sick and the doctors didn't know if nutrition, dialysis, and physical therapy would help him. At that point, it didn't matter to them. He no longer was resigned from life.

When he was finally discharged, I felt proud of the growth he had made, and I told him. He was frequently hospitalized for treatment of various infections or congestive heart failure. The night he died, his wife was at his bedside. He signed "do not resuscitate" papers. Shortly before he died, I told him that no matter how sick or healthy he was, he had already made the major leagues, and no one could ever pull him from the lineup.

EASING THE PATIENT'S HELPLESSNESS
by Elena Hanabarger (Florida, USA)

"Jack" seemed to have endless anomalies, from his cardiac dysrhythmias to his abnormal arterial blood gases (ABGs). His laboratory results were horrible—many of them incompatible with life. As I took his history, I realized that despite his obvious physical frailty, his pain originated elsewhere. He had lost his wife to cancer about a year before, and he had exhausted their savings paying for her care and treatments. After she died, he reverted to alcohol use, which he had overcome nearly 10 years prior. Suffering financial devastation, he lost his home and all his assets. He had no children, no siblings, and no living parents. He was, as I have never been, alone. He simply gave up and "crawled into the bottle." My heart ached for this man, more so than it had for any person before him. I felt sorry that he had been dealt such a devastating series of blows. I felt angry that he had to endure this pain alone, and I felt embarrassed that he was the subject of such great amusement to so many that day in the department.

I wondered why he was so abhorred. Was it his choice? Was it his appearance? Was it his attitude? Then it occurred to me. We can't fix him. We can ask him not to take another drink, we can ask him to stop mourning the loss of his beloved, we can ask him to go to a shelter rather than live under a bridge, we can ask him to brush his teeth and clean the filth from his skin—but we can't make him do any of these things. We can't force anyone against his or her will. Then suddenly it occurred to me: "will." He had no will to survive. He was not looking to overcome unbeatable odds; he wasn't trying to "beat" some disease he'd been afflicted with; he didn't even care if he was warm or cold, or if he had been fed. His only interest was finding some way to treat his "pain," be it through alcohol or a visit to the emergency department.

I remember, as I walked out of the department to go to lunch, the contrast of this dark creature resting on the stark white sheets. I remember watching him rest as we made our desperate attempts to rehydrate him. I remember, as I walked through the door, hearing chuckles and finding myself feeling sorry—but not for Jack. At lunch with a fellow nurse, I couldn't escape my thoughts of Jack. We talked about him the whole time. I wondered what he had last eaten and when that might have been. I did not pity Jack. His choices were his own. I could not judge him for what he had done or how he had lived. I wished I could think of some way to heal him; I wished there was something I could do.

When I got back, I immediately checked on him, and I decided to try something innovative. I asked him what I could do for him. Many times in nursing, we are so preoccupied with carrying out orders and telling patients what we expect of them that we forget to ask what they want or expect. He paused for a moment, and then he bravely asked if there was any way he could get a shower. He admitted to taking a shower almost a month ago, but "the water was ice cold." I remember thinking, "A shower? That's all?" I decided this would be the best shower I had ever given, and it would be the best one he'd ever had.

I collected towels, washcloths, and a specialty shower chair the water could flow through. I came back and told him that he could take a shower, and he looked at me with such an expression of gratitude. As I wheeled him into the steam-filled room, his eyes lit up at the prospect of a warm shower. As soon as the hot water touched his skin, he reached his hands up as if to embrace each drop, and he began to cry. He asked if I could just leave him there for a while, and I did. After about 10 minutes, I came back to find him still reveling in the magic of the shower. I took a cloth and began to wash him. As layer upon layer of filth rinsed clean and down the drain, his whole posture changed. The burdens of his life and lifestyle appeared to lift. After he was clean and rinsed, I turned the water off and handed him a towel. I helped him dry off and put him in a clean gown. Then I took him into the hall where his stretcher waited. I helped him onto the clean white sheets, and I tucked him under fresh, warm blankets.

As nurses, we want to fix and heal. We sometimes forget that we are more than a physical creature. We acknowledge that human beings are more than the sum of their collective organs, tissues, and cells. But do we practice as though we believe that? Do we truly search to heal the soul or spirit of our patients? In Jack's case, his spirit suffered the greatest affliction, and his pain resided in his soul.

As I left that day, I leaned over his bed. He took my hand and squeezed it ever so gently. With a look I'll never forget, he thanked me for "caring" for him.

That day forever shaped the way I practice nursing. Each day and each series of moments provide us with distinct opportunities to effect change. Just for a moment, I helped this man escape his pain, shame, and helplessness and perhaps made him feel valuable and purposeful. I bring this commitment and philosophy with me to each patient's bedside, and I hope that I never take for granted how wonderful a hot shower feels.

The words written by Elena in the previous story convey much meaning: "Just for a moment, I helped this man escape his pain, shame, and helplessness." We can't fix many of the problems patients have. We can't make choices for them. What we can do, however, is make the moments we work with the patient gratifying, respectful, and purposeful. We can ease the frustration and helplessness that patients feel. We know the ways that lead to trust and distrust. Time to heal, time to care, and a passionate commitment to the patient make the moments that matter. Let us, as nurses, never forget the purpose of our work is to care for patients, no matter the circumstance that brought them to us.

CARING BY GIVING MOMENTS THAT COUNT
by Timothy Bartell (Utah, USA)

As a new nurse, I worked in a long-term care center, which can be very challenging. I started working the minute I got there and continued working the 8-hour shift until the end, without any breaks. Patient census was always high. Most of the time, I had 20 to 50 patients. This left very little time for individual patient care and the attention many of these residents needed. There was one particular resident who stood out. I will call her Ruth.

During the latter part of Ruth's life, she had several battles with cancer. Until the last few months of her life, she had won those battles. Finally, the cancer-fighting drugs seemed no longer to work. She lost an unbelievable amount of weight as the cancer started to spread. She also lost nearly all of her ability to function. Eventually, all her activities of daily living (ADLs) were provided by nurses and certified nurse aides (CNAs).

Her physical condition made it impossible for her to remain in the same position for extended periods of time. She would ask for help with positioning every time someone entered the room. Many of the facility staff became very impatient with her, especially when she requested help only minutes after receiving it. Often, CNAs complained about having to work with Ruth because of her constant requests for attention.

I felt a lot of compassion for Ruth since I had lost a close relative to cancer. As I watched the impact of cancer on Ruth, I remembered the discomfort my relative had experienced. I decided that whenever possible, I would take the time to help Ruth reposition and get more comfortable. Each time I would do so, she would take my hand and offer a sincere, heartfelt thank you. At the time, I did not consider the significance of those expressions of gratitude.

Her husband had died many years earlier, leaving her with two young sons to raise on her own. She worked hard to raise and provide for her children. She remained spiritually strong all of her life and taught her sons to follow her example. Now, this strong, independent woman was not able to do anything for herself. I tried to imagine what it would be like to have been active and independent all of my life and now to be unable to do anything for myself. I tried to imagine the frustration she must have felt because of her helplessness.

In her final days, she was hardly able to swallow. We struggled to get her to eat or drink anything. Her doctor stopped her regular medications and ordered medication only for comfort measures.

The night before she died was very busy. I went to her room and tried to help her drink a small amount of supplement. I worked with her for a few minutes and then repositioned her. Just as I was about to leave, she took my hand and kissed it, looked into my eyes, and offered the most sincere thank you I have ever heard. I bent down and told her what a great person she was and that she had led a great life. Somehow

I knew this would be the last time I would see Ruth alive, and I believe she knew it too.

There were never any heroics in my actions. In the end, it was a little bit of extra time that mattered. Though I often spent only moments with her, those moments not only increased her comfort, but also showed her that someone cared. Let us, as nurses, never forget that it is often effort "outside what is expected" that matters most to our patients.

Giving Love
by Carolyn Sutherland (Utah, USA)

He was 28, and his name was Matt—the same age and name as my oldest son. His marrow had failed him. He didn't know it yet, but I did. He came to the oncology floor in the late afternoon, and I got him settled in, did an assessment, and visited with him briefly. Blood samples previously drawn in the emergency room (ER) were reported on the computer, and it was pretty clear Matt had leukemia.

The doctor came in to do a bone marrow biopsy. They're never pleasant. I had pushed some Demerol through his IV a few minutes before, but Demerol doesn't really take care of the bone pain. I offered my hand "to hang on to, if you need it." He didn't. He was quiet, somewhat relaxed, and independent. The procedure didn't take long. The doctor was quick, precise, and efficient. He palpated, mapped the spot with an indentation of his fingernail, cleansed the skin, and deadened the superficial tissues and then the deeper ones. The bone-coring biopsy needle slid through the tissues and then bored through the bone. A series of twists to the right was followed by a series of twists to the left to free the slender core of bone. Specimens of bone and of marrow were extracted and deftly deposited on slides. Matt pushed his face into the pillow and gripped the bed but kept his hand away from mine. A pressure dressing was applied, and Matt turned onto his back to increase the pressure on the dressing.

Now he just had to wait until tomorrow for the biopsy results to confirm what the lab report had already indicated. This one last day Matt was free from the knowledge of his diagnosis. It was Valentine's Day, and his wife, Jill, was at work and would come later with their 3-year-old daughter. For now, he was alone with his thoughts.

Matt was quiet and seldom talked about his feelings. He was, however, always courteous, and he rarely complained. We talked that afternoon about peripheral things—what had made him decide to come to the hospital, how he liked to play basketball with his friends, what he did for a living. But cutting through the insignificant details of our conversation came the gloomy thought, "I'm going to have to watch you die!"

What was that all about? I love working with oncology patients, and I'm the most optimistic oncology nurse I know. I believe every patient I work with is going to be in that percentage, however small, of patients who respond to treatment. I always tell the truth to patients, but I also help them reach for the very best outcomes possible. I pushed the thought aside and went on about my work, but I couldn't forget the feeling that had accompanied those words as they passed through my mind.

Matt had a brother whose marrow was a good match. Matt would have chemotherapy to get his leukemia in remission. After his blood counts returned to normal levels, he would come in for the bone marrow transplant (BMT).

The chemotherapy regimen went fairly well, and soon Matt was in remission. He went home to resume his life. Jill gave me a big hug, and

Matt grinned and shook my hand as he left the hospital. He and Jill were expecting their second child—a boy—and Matt would return for his transplant about the time the baby was due.

In no time at all, Matt was back for the BMT. It was a weekday, and Matt arrived wearing a suit and a white shirt. He and his wife had just come from the temple. It seemed a good way to start this phase of treatment. There was a remodeling project under way on the oncology unit, and Matt smiled as he mentioned that the architectural firm he worked for had drawn up the plans. He spent a few minutes chatting with workmen before going into his room.

A week or so of chemotherapy, a day or two of rest, and then total body irradiation. It was a formidable assault on his body, but Matt was young and strong. The radiation treatments made him anxious, and he generally got Ativan just prior to going down to the radiation center. One day I made the mistake of holding the Ativan because he had received some earlier in the day, and it was only ordered to be given every 6 hours. I would give it as soon as he returned from radiation, so he would get some good rest.

About 20 minutes after he left the unit, I got a call from the radiation center. Matt had become so anxious during radiation that the treatment had to be stopped. When I got to the radiation center, Matt was sitting in a wheelchair facing the wall in the waiting room. He was distressed and embarrassed. I was devastated. It was my fault. I had not planned well, and he was paying for it.

I gave Matt the Ativan and sat with him until he relaxed. Then I assured him I would stay until his treatment was finished, and I would watch him every minute on the monitor. I sat in the booth with the radiation techs and watched him as the techs talked to him over the intercom throughout the rest of the treatment. Then I took him back up to his room, where he relaxed and slept.

After the radiation was finished, we moved Matt into the sterile laminar air flow (LAF) room in the BMT unit where he would receive his new marrow and wait for his blood counts to return. The transplant was hard on him, but he survived it. He was so anxious and nauseated while in the LAF that he threw up every time he moved. Each day I put on sterile attire and went into his protective room to bathe him and change his central line dressing. Gradually his blood counts returned as his brother's marrow engrafted, and he emerged from his sterile cocoon. What a celebration we had! Now he just had to get off the total parenteral nutrition (TPN) and take enough nutrients orally so he could go home.

The day Matt went home, his wife brought a little present to me—a 5 X 7 framed paper decorated with childish paint strokes on which she had printed the words "Thanks for making our daddy all better." Matt and I hugged affectionately, and then he got into the car and was gone. I put the little framed note on my dresser, but I almost cringed as I read the words "all better" day after day.

Not many days passed, and Matt was brought back to the hospital emergency room. His bladder was bleeding (a late side effect of his chemotherapy), and he was very ill. Day after day we irrigated his bladder at a rate requiring a 2-liter bag to be changed every 30-40 minutes. If the irrigation slowed down, his catheter would clot and he would be in severe pain. Nearing the end of a 16-hour shift, I was helping Matt to get settled back in bed. With all the energy he could muster, he looked up at me and groaned the words "I'm so sorry to be doing this to you." I fought back the tears and assured him that it was I who was sorry to be doing this to him.

Miraculously the bleeding finally stopped, and Matt went home again, but he was not there long. He developed an infection and had to be readmitted. He had little in the way of physical energy to contribute to fighting the infection, and blood cultures showed the infection was caused by a formidable organism. I went to endoscopy with him one afternoon for a bronchoscopy. I slowly injected Ativan at intervals with one hand while Matt nearly squeezed the life out of my other hand. The culture results came back the next evening, and Matt sobbed as the doctor gave him the news. The infection was in his lungs, and there was almost no chance of survival.

A few days later, Matt had become disoriented, and the doctor ordered a scan. I was home with a cold that day, and Matt's nurse called to tell me they thought his infection had gone to his brain. She said she didn't think that I had could make him any sicker than he was and suggested I come in to see him. I met the family in radiology, and the radiologist confirmed the infection was now in his brain. Matt's parents had come from out of town, and his mother was trying to reconcile with him after having estranged herself from him for years.

Matt was wheeled back to his room, and his mother talked to him for nearly an hour. Then she came out of his room in horror and said she thought he was gone, and Jill hadn't had a chance to say goodbye. I took Matt's mother in another room and told her I believed Matt's spirit was still there in the room, and Jill could say all the things she wanted to say to him. Jill said it was all right because she and Matt "were okay" and it was his mother who really needed to talk to him. I was amazed at the wisdom, the peace, and the grace of this young widow. After the family left, I stayed in the room with Matt for a little while, not wanting him to be alone. There he was just as I had feared he would be 6 months before. His tormented body was now still and at peace. I drove home and put away the little framed note. I couldn't bear to look at it again.

Several of the nurses went to Matt's funeral. It was uplifting and comforting. Jill called me a few days later. She said, "I think Matt would want you to know that you fulfilled in him everything that was lacking with his mother." I never wanted to take the place of Matt's own mother, but I did love him, and I believe he helped me learn to be a better nurse.

A nurse chooses whether or not to care personally about a patient. I chose to care deeply about Matt—to love him as a son. The pain of separation is the price for choosing to love. The pain will go away, but the love is everlasting.

CARING BY OFFERING RESPECT
by Stacey Westphal (Florida, USA)

She caught my attention during "Resident at Risk" morning rounds, as she appeared to be dusting the nurse's station. Without a dust rag, she slowly was dusting every inch, unaware of what was going on around her. Tall, thin, and gray-haired, she had part of her blouse tucked in and another part hanging over her pants, peeking out beneath her sweater. She was in her own little world. I wanted so much to say "hi." I walked over to her and tried to communicate through eye contact but had no luck, as she did not acknowledge me. I gently put one of my hands on hers, feeling her pancake syrup-sticky fingers. Again, I received no feedback that she knew I was there. She eventually came to the end of the nurse's station, removed the Bath Book, and proceeded to the next nurse's station, again dusting without a cloth.

Stella was in a world of her own. Diagnosed with senile dementia, she would wander from one nurse's station to another all day long. She spoke rarely, if at all, and sometimes became violent with the staff. Over the next few days, I would stop each time I saw her to say "hi," but never received any reaction.

During shift change one afternoon, I spotted her in a wheelchair, strapped in with a Velcro fastening. She was agitated and trying very hard to free herself. The restraints, together with noise from the television and other residents, were clearly making her miserable. Even though Velcro restraints are easily removed, she could not release herself from the bondage that held her in place. I released her from the chair and removed her from the noisy room, but she was still in a state of agitation. I decided to sing "You Are My Sunshine." Suddenly, she calmed down and began to move up and down to the beat of the music. I reached her, for only a brief moment, until she began her journey from unit to unit.

When Stella became agitated, I sometimes brought her to my office. While I worked, I played old Mitch Miller sing-along tunes on my CD player. She would sit still for 10 to 20 minutes, tapping her feet to the music. There was someone inside to reach.

One day while I was sitting in the hall, Stella sat down in the chair next to me. A group of visiting family members, one of them a bald-headed woman, walked by. Stella turned to me and said, "Saves money on hair spray, doesn't she?" Stella and I broke out laughing. I couldn't believe she had uttered those words. There was someone in there trying to get out.

I received permission from her state-appointed guardian, a private social service firm, to take her on outings. First, we walked around the gardens surrounding the facility. She loved to look at the flowers. I picked some of the brightly colored hibiscus for her, and the smile on her face could light up the whole world. Next, we went on an outing to the local McDonald's. By then, she was speaking a little bit more, but not much. I ordered a caramel ice cream cup for her. While she ate, she looked at the people and cars traveling by. She began talking in sentences. The first outing was a success; she was interested in the world around her. The next outing was the zoo, where she had a wonderful time. However, I think she found more pleasure in looking at the people, especially the children, than the animals. She was smiling and interacting with the world around her. It was that day I received my first hug and kiss from her.

In small excerpts, she eventually was able to tell me about her brother and her mother. She would not speak of anyone else in her life. But Stella loved to sit and listen to stories of my family; I would tell her about all the latest family news.

The staff also noticed Stella had changed. I don't know if her behavior changed because I had reached her, or if it changed because the staff now treated her differently due to the special interest I had taken in her. I suspect it is because they now treated her differently. I would catch staff singing to her when she became agitated, and they would bring her to the afternoon music programs. She loved to dance, and staff members would dance with her. Her violent outbursts disappeared. The staff learned how to use distraction by singing.

I often told Stella she was the best hugger in the entire world. That would make her laugh and put a big smile on her face. My coworkers would ask Stella, "Who's that with you?" She would reply, "Barbara." To this day I do not think she knows my name, but when she sees me, her arms open wide and there's a smile on her face. I realize now that if you treat people as though they were institutionalized, they will fill that role. If you treat them with respect and like worthwhile individuals, they respond in kind.

CARING BY BEING A FRIEND
by Wendy J. Berg (Florida, USA)

When I first met Roberta, she was a 19-year-old pregnant woman on our high-risk obstetric unit, dealing with the risk of losing her baby. She was being treated for preterm labor at 20 weeks' gestation. I administered intravenous magnesium sulfate to stop her contractions, antibiotics to prevent infection, and steroids to speed the baby's lung maturity. Magnesium sulfate causes blurred vision and makes patients feel hot, weak, and nauseous. Confined to bed, Roberta also was attached to a fetal monitor, an oximeter, and a blood pressure cuff, with a Foley catheter draining her bladder. She faced the prospect of remaining in the hospital on bed rest for many weeks and possibly months.

I was impressed with how determined she was to do everything we suggested to improve her baby's chance for survival. In my experiences with teen mothers, they are often unable to see beyond their own wants and desires and think about what is best for their baby. Roberta seemed very mature for her 19 years, perhaps because she was already the mother of a beautiful 18-month-old boy. She desperately wanted this baby and was motivated to do anything necessary. Roberta had a limited support system in the local area. Her mother and sisters lived in another state. She lived with her boyfriend and despite their young ages, they had a very caring and supportive relationship. Her boyfriend worked full time, and she spent most of her days in the hospital alone. I had many opportunities to talk with Roberta and to listen as she described her love for her son and boyfriend. I was at the bedside to offer tissues when she cried because she missed them. She also worried that she had done something to cause preterm labor. I reassured her that we often do not know why someone has preterm labor, and this was not anyone's fault.

Roberta spent approximately 2 weeks with us in the hospital, but ultimately we lost this fight. Baby Victoria was delivered at only 22 weeks gestation and did not survive. I was not working the day she delivered but heard the story 2 days later when I returned to work. Roberta had already been discharged home, and normally that would have been the end of my role as her nurse.

I received a call from Roberta only because I was the one who happened to answer the phone. She was desperately trying to contact the hospital chaplain to find a minister to officiate at Baby Victoria's funeral. I could have just given her the phone number for the hospital chaplain, but she wanted to talk. As I listened, she began to cry. Her family was not able to be with her, and she was overwhelmed with the details of the funeral, the normal postpartum hormones flooding her body, and the grief over her loss. She still worried that something she had done had caused Baby Victoria to be born too early. When she told me the funeral was scheduled for the next day, New Year's Eve, I listened to my heart and asked her if she would like me to be there. She said yes and became calmer.

That phone call made a difference in this woman's life and my life. So often, nursing care keeps us too busy to really hear the needs of our patients. Roberta didn't really need a nurse. She needed a friend. She needed her mother. She needed someone who recognized the significance of her loss. In my role as a nurse, I just happened to be the one to answer that phone. I happened to be there to share her feelings. Fortunately, I was not too busy that day to really hear and be her friend.

My 10-year-old daughter accompanied me to the cemetery. We brought gifts. I brought Roberta a book about grieving and loss, and my daughter brought a soft little lamb for Baby Victoria. I waited in the car for family and friends to arrive, planning to blend in with the crowd. But, a lone car with Roberta and her boyfriend pulled up to the gravesite. We gave hugs, our gifts, and our words of condolences. Tears were already streaming down her face. Nobody else ever arrived for the funeral.

Baby Victoria's tiny casket was brought out to the gravesite. The minister spoke words of comfort as Roberta's tears gave way to weeping. At the end of the ceremony, she threw herself on the little casket, and her body shook with violent sobs. Her boyfriend seemed overwhelmed by her emotions and remained in his seat. After a few moments, I walked up and put my arm around her. She turned to me, and I held her as she rocked back and forth crying. Together we cried for Baby Victoria, and I cried for all the babies I had seen born too early. We stayed until they asked us to move in order to fill the grave. Roberta asked them to wait as she put the Beanie Baby lamb on top of the coffin. Then shovels of dirt were poured over Baby Victoria and her lamb.

I was appalled that none of her friends and family made the trip to the cemetery that day. The impression I received from Roberta was that everyone seemed to think losing a baby this early was no big deal. She was told to get over it and move on with her life. No recognition was given to her need to grieve over this great loss.

I ran into Roberta a few months later, and she was doing well. This story does have a happier ending. When I last saw Roberta, she was being admitted to the hospital with a 9-months-pregnant belly. She gave me a hug and told me she and her boyfriend had married, and their son was now 3 years old. At this stay at our hospital, she delivered another healthy baby boy. Roberta and her husband hope to be back to have a baby girl in the not-too-distant future.

Nursing has granted me the privilege of intimately touching and being touched by the lives of those entrusted into my care. I am grateful for a profession that allows me to really make a difference in the lives of others.

MAKING TIME TO LISTEN
by Alzebeta Hanzlikova (Slovak Republic)

I worked in the preoperative room of a well-known hospital. The surgeons conducted thoracic operations on patients who came from all regions of the country. One night on my shift, an older patient with cancer could not sleep and wanted to talk to me. In the room were six patients. All the patients slept except for my patient, who was awake. He spoke to me about his life, his family, and his children. I was very young, but I felt he needed me for support. The next morning I went home. I came in to work the next shift, and my patient was not in the bed; he had died. I was very sad but felt satisfied about the care I had given him. Several days later, a younger woman and older woman came to see me. They were the wife and daughter of my patient. They had heard I was the last person to be with him. They needed my support and were very grateful that I had time to talk with them. Even today, I see the eyes of that patient, and I have not forgotten him. Perhaps that is the reason I fight for higher education for nurses and for change in our profession. That day is over, but patient-focused nursing remains important.

CARING BY REMOVING FEARS
by Nancy Barnhouse (Florida, USA)

On my way to teach an orthopedic preoperative class, I thought about how the patients would just listen to me and then be on their way. While teaching the class, I noticed one lady in particular who was taking notes. She was one of the few who asked questions. As I started cleaning up at the end of class, the woman called me by name. She said "Nancy, do you have a moment?" I said, "Of course." I pulled up a chair next to her and asked how I could help. She said, "This probably sounds dumb, but I'm scared." I noticed true fear in her eyes and a crack in her voice. I reached for her hand as she started to cry. I sat silently for a few moments, pondering my next choice of words. "It's all right" or "I understand" just didn't seem like the right words. So I said, "I've never had surgery, but I deal with patients on a daily basis who have had surgery like yours. I want you to leave here confident and unafraid, no matter how long it takes." I gave her a tissue and some water and sat back down with her. She started to tell me that she was most afraid of "things that can go wrong after surgery." I explained to her in precise detail the post-op plans and routines for patients who were having a total joint replacement. Pain and mobility impairment were among her biggest fears. Knowing which physician was going to perform her surgery, I knew that she would return with a morphine PCA pump at default settings and no basal rate. I explained to her exactly what that meant. I told her the pain button would deliver her pain medicine. She was happy that she had control. She explained that she thought the nurses would "not give me enough pain medicine to keep me comfortable." I explained the purpose of the basal rate and warned her she would not have a continuous infusion of morphine. But I reassured her that if the settings ordered for her were not helping, she could ask the nurse to call the doctor. She was much more at ease knowing she had these options.

Then she spoke of mobility impairment. She was certain she was going to lose independence. "I don't want to be a burden," she said. Again, I ran through the precautions after a total hip arthroplasty. But this time it felt different. I was not "teaching" or "explaining"; I was giving hope and lifting her burden. After about an hour we departed. "Mrs. K." was satisfied, and I was fulfilled.

I think someone was watching her the week of surgery. I was on duty, scheduled to work three 12-hour shifts in a row. I was assigned to a post-op total hip arthroplasty in room 822; it was Mrs. K. I knew she would be thrilled to see me, and I hoped she remembered me. Her surgery went fine, with no complications. As her bed was rolled into her room, her husband saw me and smiled. Mrs. K. had her eyes closed. I spoke to her. She opened her eyes wide, looked at me, and searched for my hand. She said, "God bless you child, for all you've done for me." I smiled and said, "You're welcome. Now let's start healing."

She was doing well. Her pain was under control. She was using her PCA, and it was extremely effective. I had the pleasure of being her nurse for 3 days. By the third day, she was ambulating about 75-100 feet. She was discharged to a rehabilitation facility. As she was leaving, she thanked me again. I told her that she was the one who did a good job. After she left, I realized that I do make a true difference in my patients' lives. No matter how small it seems to me, it could mean the world to others.

The true appreciation of this story came 3 months later. I was working one afternoon when one of my coworkers asked me if I would see a patient who was asking for me. Baffled, I wondered who it could be. As I entered the room, I saw Mrs. K. My heart sank. The first thing that came to mind was dislocation or infection. I pulled a chair next to hers. She smiled and reached for my hand. My first question was, "What happened?" She smiled and told me, "I had such a wonderful experience with your help the first time, I thought I'd try the other hip alone." We sat and talked a few minutes. I was called to attend to another patient. As I left, she told me she was being discharged. Again, I wished her luck. She said, "If it wasn't for you talking with me at class, I would never have had this done, much less both my hips. Now I can live out the rest of my life without disease or pain. Thank you."

I truly did make a difference in someone's life that day. For Mrs. K., this influence will be with her for the rest of her life. I hope to be there for all my patients. I am truly blessed to be a nurse.

CARING BY LIFTING A BURDEN
by Barbara T. Lorenz (Florida, USA)

Have you ever become so fixated on the complexity of the disease process and the technical nursing skills needed to care for a patient that you minimize the psychosocial impact of your nursing actions? The answer to this question is "yes" for me, and a particular patient comes to mind—a 34-year-old woman with multiple complications resulting from an inherited disease, cystic fibrosis. She suffered end-stage lung disease with subsequent lung transplantation, severe peripheral vascular disease, and end-stage renal failure secondary to immuno-suppressive agents required after transplantation. Statistically speaking, she had already surpassed the 30-year life expectancy for cystic fibrosis patients.

She was my first patient with this diagnosis. I was a new nurse practitioner on a recently opened acute care unit. Upon entering her room, I observed a petite, frail, and courageous young woman whose smile and sense of humor quickly melted away the anxieties I had about caring for a patient with such complex diagnoses. After examining her, I realized this would not be a simple case, and the likelihood of a favorable outcome was slim. At that moment, I wondered if a patient this seriously ill was more than my nursing skills could handle.

My patient had learned at an early age to be in control and participate in her healthcare. An organized person, she always had questions about her medical care, using old envelopes or the tops of tissue boxes to jot down small details lest she forget them. Often the last words uttered before I exited the room were, "Oh, one more thing ..." I felt quite inept because I could not provide answers to many of her questions, but she seemed pleased that I would diligently seek all explanations possible to the questions.

She was hospitalized countless times during the last year of her life, spiraling downward toward progressively worse prognoses. Each setback weighed heavily on my mind and even more heavily on my heart. My mood would often revolve around the bad news I had to break to her and her supportive family members. She endured several painful operative procedures, including below-the-knee amputations to ease excruciating neurogenic pain and nonhealing wounds. On her last admission to our facility, she once again was faced with the decision to amputate a finger. At that moment, I sensed that she had already made up her mind to follow a different path, one that would lead to the end of the pain and suffering she had endured during her life.

She deferred her decision for further surgery and decided to return home. It was no surprise to me to learn that she had contacted hospice services to assist and comfort her during her dying process. She did, however, choose to continue dialysis temporarily in an effort to gain additional time to complete some unfinished business. Shortly before her death, her mother visited our unit carrying a large bouquet of fresh flowers with a note attached. This selfless act by her mother was most courageous, as her mother knew that she would soon have to endure the loss of her third child to the ravages of cystic fibrosis. The attached note thanked all the nurses who cared for and supported her and her family during those difficult times. It was strange. For a second I thought I heard a voice saying, "Oh, one more thing ..." Perhaps thanking us was one small part of her unfinished business.

A few days later, we learned that she had died and that with the help of hospice, she was quite comfortable in the end. I was relieved to know her pain and suffering had ended, but there remained an unsettled feeling I could not shake. Each day for nearly a week, I walked past the bouquet of flowers and asked myself, "Did I really fulfill all of her and her family's needs, both physically and emotionally?" Without a doubt, advanced medical technologies, medicines, and nursing care had brought this patient well past her life expectancy. And if in the days prior to her death, taking the time to complete part of her unfinished business was affirmation that our caring and support during her life and death did not go unnoticed, then the answer to this question is "yes" for me.

"The lessons I learned were invaluable." Nurses say these words each day. Nurses learn that things they thought could never be accomplished happen anyway because of their deep caring. Just because it was "never done that way before," the nurse gets it done. Just because they are told "no" by another healthcare worker, it doesn't mean they won't get their way. Nurses are leaders, not followers. They lead the family, the healthcare team, and other nurses. They are the glue that bonds an organization together.

Nurses befriend patients by making valentines for them and decorating their rooms to change the scenery and uplift their spirits. Sometimes nurses just talk with patients about "stuff"... a car, a motorcycle, how to play blackjack. At other times, they give keen attention to patients who want to share their families' activities or their personal accomplishments. They truly help patients find closure and a sense of completion in their lives. You cannot put a price tag on this level of concern and caring. The power and dedication of nurses, and their emotional and spiritual strength in times of adversity, are common in the workday of the nurse.

CARING BY HONORING SPIRITUAL STRENGTH
by Kent D. Blad (Utah, USA)

"Mr. P." was a 70-year-old veteran of World War II. He came to our hospital in need of treatment for recently diagnosed cancer of the esophagus. After discussion with the family and physicians, the decision was made to take the patient to surgery to perform an esophagogastrectomy. Upon completion of his surgery, Mr. P. returned to the surgical intensive care unit (SICU) for his postoperative care. Mr. P.'s wife and children spent many hours at his bedside, holding hands, praying, and offering words of encouragement to their recovering husband and father. With joy and smiles, they witnessed his seemingly uneventful wakening from anesthesia and recovery in those first few days following surgery. Mr. P. was a delightful, pleasant individual who shared his love for his family and expressed his appreciation for their support.

Mr. P.'s condition held steady for less than a week in the SICU. He began to have trouble with his tube feedings and complained of nausea and vomiting, abdominal pain, and not feeling well. The decision was made to discontinue his tube feedings and begin total parenteral nutrition through his intravenous (IV) catheter. After a week's trial of this and other treatments, Mr. P.'s condition worsened. The family shared their concerns with the physician and staff, as they worried about his unusual behavior.

During those weeks of caring for Mr. P. and his family, I, as his primary nurse, became very emotionally attached to them. I found myself spending more and more time in the room at the patient's bedside, trying to do everything possible. I found my efforts were not helping Mr. P. with his recovery. The family and I were concerned that Mr. P.'s lack of improvement might indicate a serious problem. The concerns were relayed to the surgical team, followed by a lengthy discussion with the family on the best treatment to pursue. A decision was made to take Mr. P. back to surgery to explore the possible causes of his pain and lack of improvement.

In surgery, the surgeons discovered Mr. P. had a new problem, coupled with his battle with cancer. The tissue around the operative sight had eroded, causing the tissue to tear, which in turn caused his tube feedings to leak into the surrounding area. With such fragile tissue, the possibility of closing the tear was questionable. In addition, his primary esophageal cancer had metastasized. Mr. P.'s surgery was completed, unsuccessfully, and he was returned to his SICU room.

The surgical team shared the findings with the family, with the outlook of an estimated one-week survival for Mr. P. The shock of the news saddened the family. The rest of that day was spent grieving and trying to accept the facts that had been presented. The family returned home that evening to consider their options with Mr. P.'s care.

When the family returned to the hospital the next day, they proposed they take Mr. P. home to grant his wish of dying at home. My immediate reaction was, "We can't do that; that's never been done before. He needs us to take care of him." I couldn't see past his need for dressing changes, pain medication, oxygen, a hospital bed, etc.

Over the following hour or so, I thought intently about the family's request. I started questioning my response to them. Why couldn't they take him home? Why couldn't we teach the family the necessary tasks to care for him at home? Just because it had never been done before, was that enough reason for not trying? If this were my spouse or father, would I want his wish granted? I became convinced this was not an impossible task. We were going to take Mr. P. home.

The wheels started spinning. I wanted to support Mr. P's wishes, and I shared this with the family. I told them about our slim odds of being able to accomplish this, but at least we were willing to give it our best shot. The first hurdle was to get the surgical team to agree. After their evaluations of Mr. P. and discussions of our plans, the surgical team gave permission for us to start the process as soon as possible. Confirming orders were written to allow for Mr. P.'s release. The next hours were spent arranging for the necessary equipment to be delivered to the home. In coordination with home healthcare, a hospital bed, wound dressing supplies, morphine, and oxygen, as well as many other items, were scheduled to be delivered to the home the next morning. Since time was of the essence, transportation was arranged to take him home at the beginning of the next day. The final few hours of that day were spent teaching his wife and children the tasks of changing dressings, administering the medication and oxygen administration, and so on.

The next morning, I arrived before the family, visited with Mr. P., and shared with him the excitement the day would bring for him and his family. With limited energy, he continued to smile throughout our conversation. His dream was going to come true. I hastily made a sign to put near him. As his family arrived, they read, "PLEASE TAKE ME HOME!"

The memory of that moment when the family entered the room, prepared to take their loved one home, will forever be imprinted on my mind. In spite of the tragic circumstances surrounding the situation, I will never forget the look of love, appreciation, and joy on their faces. The emotions shared were not ones of sadness, but happiness. This good, kind gentleman was now free to go home and die with dignity and peace, with his loving family surrounding him.

Word came from the family that Mr. P. died on the third day after returning home, with a smile on his face and his entire family surrounding his bed. The lessons I learned were invaluable. Things could be accomplished that hadn't been done before. I learned the power of dedication and emotional and spiritual strength during times of adversity. I will never be the same, nor will I ever approach a patient in the same manner as I did before caring for Mr. P.

Can caring really be taught? Or is it just part of someone's nature? The following exemplar focuses on Patricia Benner's (1984) domain of nursing practice, "the healing relationship." Nurse Terri O'Brien creates a climate for and a commitment to healing. For Mr. and Mrs. T. and their 15-year-old son, she personifies hope, finds an acceptable understanding of a very serious situation, and provides a teaching plan the entire family can follow effectively. She makes the best out of an extremely wobbly situation.

CARING BY BEING A PATIENT TEACHER
by Terri O'Brien (Florida, USA)

On Nov. 29, "Mrs. T." entered the emergency room with a history of 3 days' shortness of breath and a productive cough. She was admitted to the intermediate intensive care unit (MICU) with acute respiratory insufficiency and acute lung injury from community acquired pneumonia. Her blood cultures were positive for pseudomonas and staphylococcus. By Dec. 2, she had persistent ventilator dependency with a declining respiratory situation on 100% oxygen.

After 28 days on a ventilator, Mrs. T. was finally extubated. However, all was not well. She was extremely lethargic and had profound muscular weakness consistent with polyneuropathy. She showed significant motor weakness and lethargy. A psychiatric consult revealed possible catatonic depression with a severe anxiety component. Finally, an electroencephalogram (EEG) revealed moderately diffuse, slowly predominate waves over the frontal areas of the brain with prior global injury in the form of septic encephalopathy. Apparently, at some point over the last month, the sepsis had spread to her brain and caused encephalitis.

On Jan. 3, she was transferred to a medical unit. However, after only 2 days, she experienced increasing respiratory distress and anxiety. She was transferred back to MICU with recurrent hypoglycemia, a worsening mental attitude, and changes in her bilateral chest X-ray. She was reintubated. From what I understand about acute respiratory distress syndrome (ARDS), a reoccurrence is not that unusual. She remained intubated until Jan. 19, another 14 days. Her affect remained flat. Finally, after a hospitalization of 66 days, she was transferred to a rehabilitation center.

To make matters worse, Mrs. T. had one other medical problem to add to her long list. She was 32 weeks' pregnant when she first came into the hospital. Her baby wasn't due until Jan. 21. On Dec. 2, the decision to perform a C-section was made because of Mrs. T.'s declining respiratory status. At birth, "Baby A" was floppy with no spontaneous respirations, due to maternal anesthesia. She was intubated and given Narcan, with limited response. Her Apgar scores were 3 and 5, and she was immediately transferred to the neonatal intensive care unit (NICU). Her initial diagnosis included respiratory distress syndrome (RDS), for which she received Survanta; hypoglycemia, for which she received a bolus of IV fluids; presumed sepsis, due to the mother's positive cultures of pseudomonas and staphylococcus, for which she received antibiotics; hypotension, requiring a dopamine/dobutamine drip for 2 days; a two-vessel cord, which meant she could have renal anomalies; and a grade I intraventricular hemorrhage, which resolved by Dec. 18. Baby A remained intubated until Dec. 6 and on oxygen until Dec. 12. After 7 days of antibiotics, her cultures revealed no sepsis. She began nasal tube feedings on Dec. 7 and was taking fluids by mouth within 7 days. On Dec. 27, at 25 days of age, she was discharged to her father.

I know Baby A received exemplary care, and I'm quite sure her mother did also. This story is not about them or their care, as any competent ICU nurse could have cared for these two patients. The clinical information was necessary to relate, however, because it provides the background for the circumstances facing Mrs. T's husband and Baby A.

My story is about teaching a new father total infant care. Normally, we teach the mother infant care, and sometimes the father will feed the baby, change diapers, or give baths. This particular father had to deal with his wife being critically ill in MICU while his daughter was critically ill in NICU. The poor man was torn between the two. Whom should he visit first? Whom should he stay with? Who needed him the most? Neither one could interact with him initially, as his wife was heavily sedated on a ventilator and Baby A was still drugged from her mother's sedation.

Baby A gradually improved, and the sedation wore off. Now there was some hope, something for Baby A's father to see as improvement in at least one of the patients. Every time I was on duty and every time he visited, we talked about the progress of both his wife and baby. I dreaded hearing his reports about his wife, as they were usually pretty negative and hopes for her recovery were dim. I gave him an opportunity to express his feelings and concerns and share his problems. I provided a listening ear and attempted to support him emotionally. These interactions took a lot of time, and I tried hard not to let him know I had a million other things to do. Thank God for my supportive coworkers, who were there when I needed a hand with my other patients. Slowly his focus turned toward Baby A. When I saw his readiness and willingness to learn, I gradually introduced him to her care. His only other child, a son, was 15, so holding, feeding, bathing, changing diapers, and dressing an infant were mostly new to him. And, to make matters worse, she was a tiny, delicate preemie. We took it a day at a time. I spent hours talking to him, teaching him, and reassuring him he was doing great. We normally take this type of teaching interaction for granted with mothers, because the maternal instinct usually takes over and our job is easier. We tried to talk about his wife in a very positive manner, but also about what he would do if the baby were discharged without her.

He was a terrific student, perhaps better than some of the mothers I've taught, so my job became quite easy. He also had a helper. His 15-year-old son learned her care right along with Dad. A nicer, more compassionate, and caring young man I've never met. Toward the end of their stay, Dad or big brother would come into the unit, take over all of Baby A's care, and spend hours cuddling and holding her. They were as comfortable with her as we were with them. A distinct bond had formed among all of us. Then it was Christmas. How sad to have to spend it in the hospital, but how happy everyone was. Baby A was going home in 2 days, and her mother was extubated for the first time the day after Christmas. We celebrated with them and included them in the unit's festivities. We took the bonding effort one step further—we took Baby A to see her mom every opportunity we had, a gesture we feel may have contributed to her recovery.

Unfortunately, all was not well. The father's only support system in the area was his wife's family—a mother and a sister. Initially, they blamed him for Mrs. T.'s illness and ensuing problems. They refused to help him care for the baby after discharge unless they could have her all the time. Actually, this may have been a blessing in disguise. The father was determined to prove he could care for his baby girl, the mother's 7-year-old child from a previous marriage, his own son, and hold down a job. How he did it, I'll never know. We were in constant communication with social services, who arranged all the community support that was available. Finally, perhaps because of his noble efforts, the family came together, learned CPR, and Baby A was discharged on Dec. 26.

On Feb. 1, when I came to work, Baby A and her big brother were waiting for me in the lobby. Mom was going to be discharged the next day, and they had come to see me for the last time. Baby A was up to 7 pounds and looked great. The surge of pride I felt when I saw them and their smiles, and their happiness at seeing me, made me realize I had actually helped to make a difference in their lives. Our purpose statement in NICU includes not only providing a nurturing environment for optimal patient outcomes, but also being an advocate for patients and their families in all (and that's a big all) aspects of care.

What is fascinating in the stories written by nurses is that many do not view their work as extraordinary. It is what they do each day. It is part of the day, part of the profession. Sometimes, in writing the story, even years later, nurses recognize experiences that have left a mark on their lives. Some have burned a memory so deep it is difficult to bear. Some have had experiences they will never forget, ones that have changed their lives and sometimes their career paths.

Putting pen to paper, nurses express profound relief, catharsis, and freedom—freedom to move on, with no regrets. The emotional toll of these experiences has been heavy, but in writing them down the nurses can sometimes lift their heavy burdens.

Are others in nursing feeling the same need to journal their caring practices? Has journaling past experiences been therapeutic to the nurse? In doing so, nurses have discovered inner feelings they didn't know they had about their profession. The tremendous courage and enormous giving of themselves, their hearts, and their minds is worthy of much praise. The writings have allowed them to develop both spiritually and emotionally. The writings have alleviated pain and left a sense of accomplishment, career validation, and appreciation for the tremendous contributions they have made to the care of their patients.

REFERENCES

Benner, P. (1984). From novice to expert: Excellence and power in clinical nursing practice. California: Addison-Wesley.

Krathwohl, D.R., Bloom, B.S., & Masia, B.B. (1964). Taxonomy of education objectives: The classification of educational goals. Handbook 2: Affective domain. New York: Longmont.

Scotto, C. (2003). A new view of caring. Journal of Nursing Education, 42(7), 289.

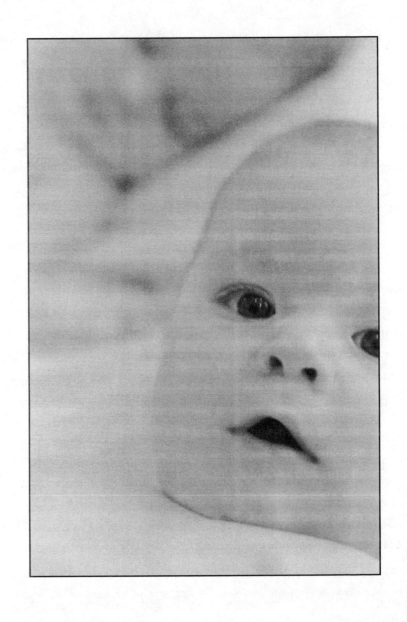

CHAPTER 3

Being Compassionate: When Special Actions Are Needed

Caring for women and children takes special skills. Some nurses say this type of nursing actually requires becoming family for awhile. You give so much of your best nursing skills and interpersonal communication techniques trying to make often terrible situations a little better. Nurses get to know everything about a child patient—favorite colors, favorite pizza, favorite ice cream, an e-mail address, or even the statistics of a favorite basketball team. Nurses clumsily sing Britney Spears' songs and French braid ponytails. Sometimes the hair is gone but other measures are taken—baseball caps and stylish dude scarves must do on certain days of the chemo cycles. Thumbs-up, a three-step handshake, dancing in the halls, nurses are at their "coolest" when adapting the trendy habits and mannerisms of youth. Their goals are to keep it all going, in a light, humorous, yet appropriate, manner for their young patients.

Gently, and oh-so-carefully, wrapping a newborn; cleansing the vernix; and placing the child in the arms of a loving mother—nurses are there. When beautiful twins are born, nurses are there. When organ donation paperwork is filed, with a grieving family in the next room, nurses are there. When hope is offered, when a new birth is celebrated, when honest words of encouragement are needed when a stillborn baby is lying in its mother's arms—nurses are always there.

Their skills are excellent as they insert feeding tubes through miniature nostrils or insert tubes in little arms barely the width of pretzel sticks. Nurses are completely in control; timing every respiration and monitoring for meconium stained fluid, the nurse is the calm in some very stormy waters. Children and babies are all treated equally, and nurses are there for the duration—morning, noon, night, and every day and every moment caring for families.

Caring for families is a roller coaster of emotions. Family dynamics can be harsh and often unruly. How do you comfort a 17-year-old mother who had delivered a baby because of rape—and still worse—that her father raped her? How do you even begin to communicate with this young woman who is wearing a necklace of bad memories that you can never even imagine! Nurses find a way. Their work with families is healing and spiritual—prayer and love for a patient is often a significant part of their care. Family nursing is immensely rewarding, in spite of the many wicked turns that keep nurses on their toes.

Professionally, family nursing is a well-defined specialty. It is the cornerstone of caring for women and children. Family-centered nursing includes childbearing and childrearing. The family could be nuclear: mother, father, and child (Pillitteri, 1999), or it could simply be a mother and child, or even an older brother caring for the little ones.

Nurse practitioners and midwives provide care to childbearing mothers. These advanced practice nurses are extraordinary caregivers.

Their assessment skills and years of clinical experience ensure safe births, extensive discharge planning, and quality teaching programs. They also work with seriously ill children, reassuring and teaching families. Nurses evaluate nursing interventions for parents and children (Santacroce, 2003). Their work in the community with families is unsurpassed. The community is often a remote location where children desperately need nursing care, where they suffer from a wide range of physical needs, such as vitamin deficiencies, malnutrition, diarrhea, or acute respiratory infections (Grubesic & Selwyn, 2003). In many community settings, the nurse is the only caregiver. You find them in underserved areas. Nurses work in not-for-profit primary care clinics that are even open on the weekends. These clinics ensure that care is provided to families (Hartley, 2002).

The family could be multigenerational and extended, including grandmothers, aunts, and cousins. Whatever comprises the family, nurses often deal with families in crisis. Their jobs include empowering the family to survive the current stress, or teaching parents to accept what often can't be changed. They assist family members to verbalize personal reactions and help them to reach out for support in the community. Nurses help families to face difficult situations with honesty and strength.

The family with an ill child probably is the most challenging of all nursing responsibilities. What do you do when your next admission is exactly the same age as your son? What, in fact, if the child is your son's classmate, or even a relative. What do you do when the parents hear that six-letter word: C-A-N-C-E-R. Nurses will tell you that every single aspect of their beings is given to these families. See how nurses open their arms—and hearts—to care for the men, women, babies, and children who cross their paths in family nursing.

COPING WITH DEATH
by Tyrone Brown (North Carolina, USA)

We often think of the nurse as the one who has "the healer's art," but on this particular day it was two patients who touched my heart. Three years ago my life plan took a dramatic change. I was a football player for Brigham Young University, a nationally ranked Division I team. Like many players, I had the dream of playing in the National Football League. During my sophomore year, I suffered an injury that caused two herniated discs in my lower back and ended my career as a football player. Not only was my dream cut short, it was obliterated completely. Despite this unfortunate event, I was a firm believer that other doors open when one door is closed.

I had a close friend who encouraged me to go into nursing. I courageously, and with an extreme alteration to my ego, acted upon his advice! I applied to and was accepted into the nursing program at Brigham Young University (BYU).

After about half a year in the program, I was going into the clinical rotation that I dreaded most: labor and delivery. This is where my story begins. You see, I'm six-foot-three, male, muscular, African American, and bald (by choice). Sometimes I see myself in the mirror and I get scared! I was terrified that the patients and other nurses would be so afraid of me, they would ask me to leave the room or wait outside the door during my time there. Most of all I thought, "How am I, a man, going to offer encouragement and support to a woman when I have no clue what it is like to be pregnant and in labor?" I thought the entire duration there was going to be miserable and a waste of time.

Ironically, this turned out not to be the case at all; it turned out to be one of my most memorable experiences as a nursing student. It was during this assignment that I had an experience that would expand my perspective and outlook on life, for it was this experience that taught me what the healer's art is all about.

On this particular day, I was assigned to work with a nurse who would be helping a mother recover physically and emotionally after giving birth to a stillborn baby that morning. When we walked in the room to introduce ourselves, a Catholic priest was there giving the baby a blessing. The baby was in the arms of a young boy who was lying down asleep on a bed. I later learned that this young boy had cried himself to sleep with his baby brother in his arms. The room was dark and smelled of blood and body fluids. The father was in the bathroom.

We learned from the night shift nurse that the father had passed out when the baby was born. The mother was lying in bed with the sheets covered in blood. She was sad, disappointed, and confused. This would have been her eighth child. She was diagnosed with chronic hypertension and had had poor prenatal care. The baby had apparently been dead for a month because upon her admission to the hospital she reported no fetal movement for about this length of time.

Finally, the priest left the room, and then the nurse also left to get a consent form so an autopsy could be performed. I was alone with this grief-stricken family. I sat beside the father as he held his baby boy in his arms. I didn't know what to say, so I didn't say anything at all. I just put my hand on his shoulder. The nurse returned to the room with the consent form. The father then asked me if I could hold the baby while he signed the papers. It was a moment in time that I will never forget. There was not the usual movement, crying, or opening of the mouth and eyes. There was blood around the baby's mouth and eyes, and on his head. Vernix was still around his arms and legs. A million thoughts rushed through my mind. I thought about what this little boy's life would have been like. I thought about all the fun things he would miss out on in life, like learning how to throw a baseball or riding a bike or having his first kiss.

The nurse and I finished helping this family. We switched the mother to another bed. We took the baby to the morgue. I learned all about the process and the extensive amount of paperwork that must be completed in these terrible situations.

Later that day as I was sitting at the nurses' station watching the fetal monitor of a new patient, one of the nurses walked by with a newborn and asked me if I would hold the baby while she finished getting a few things together. As I held this live and active newborn in my arms, I thought about my earlier experience. I could feel the heartbeat of this new baby boy. He opened his mouth wide and moved his arms and body. I couldn't help but smile and feel love for this precious gift of life. My troubled heart was beginning to mend.

The first time I held a baby in labor and delivery was when I held the stillborn. The second time was later that day when I held the live newborn. In just one day I saw and felt the whole spectrum of the good and bad.

You see, most of the time we think of the nurse as the one who has the healer's art, but on this day it was these two tiny little babies who opened my heart and touched it forever. Who knows, maybe it was part of this little stillborn's mission to come to earth and touch my life. I will never forget him. He will always remain close to my heart.

Supporting Patient Decisions
by Laura Linton (Utah, USA)

At the age of 17, Michelle conceived through a rape committed by her father. Michelle did not talk much with the nurses or her family. The night nurse suggested we care for her one-on-one so she could receive better attention and care. During the day we found out a little more about the family. Michelle discovered she was pregnant when she started to feel the baby move at about 4 months along. She tried to find out if she could have an abortion, but it was too late. Michelle finally told her mother, who was divorced from her father, when the baby was 8 months along. Together, Michelle and her mother found out about an adoption agency in Utah that would provide support and care for expectant mothers willing to give their babies up for adoption. Michelle and her mother decided it was the best thing to do, so they came to Utah for the delivery even though Michelle's mother lost her job in doing so.

Throughout the day, Michelle's mother would talk with us, yet Michelle would only say a few words. One time I went in to check on her alone, without a nurse or the girl's mother. I started joking around and tried to see how she was really doing. After a couple of minutes, Michelle started to smile and glanced at me for a second. Then a little while later she laughed a bit, made eye contact, and actually had a pleasant look on her face. Throughout the day she grew to be more comfortable with me and told me how she was feeling. She was very scared. She was in a lot of pain, not only physical, but emotional. She said that she did not want to hold the baby after the birth, but did want to see the baby. She did not want to remember this as her first child. She wanted to have a family the right way; not the way this baby had been conceived. She had a stack of letters from possible parents sitting on her bedside table. We all looked through them to see if we could help her pick out the perfect parents for the baby. She decided on one family if it was a girl and another one if it was a boy.

That afternoon Michelle delivered a very healthy, beautiful baby boy. He was perfect in every way. It was hard to believe what his mother had gone through to deliver him. We showed her the baby, asked again if she wanted to hold him. She said "no," so we took him to the nursery.

The next day, I was assigned to the postpartum unit. In report, we found out Michelle wanted to have the baby in her room during the night and then had decided to keep him. She was sobbing all night and not communicating with the nurses. Everyone was worried because the family did not have a place to live—they had been staying in shelters for the last month. Neither Michelle nor her mother had a job or any money, and they had no place to go. They would have to reimburse the adoption agency for all the services the agency had already provided and try to find a place to go after leaving the hospital. Also, Michelle did not seem emotionally prepared for such a huge responsibility. She asked to talk to a counselor to try and work things out.

Because of the time I spent with Michelle the day before and the rapport we had developed, the other nurses wanted me to care for her. I went in to find out how she was doing. Her mother was excited to see me, but Michelle wouldn't look at me and didn't answer my questions. Her mother said she had never been the type to talk to anyone and was quiet about her feelings and the issues she was dealing with.

I went back in a little bit later, sat on Michelle's bed, put my hand on hers, and said, "I heard that you had a rough night. What happened?" The tears started pouring down her face. I held her hand more tightly, waited a moment, and then quietly asked her if she wanted to keep her baby. The tears came harder, and she nodded and looked up at me and said, "Yes."

"That must be so hard to carry a baby for 9 months, see such a beautiful boy, and then give him up," I replied. She nodded. "So what are you going to do?" I asked.

She sat there for a moment, looked up at me again, and said, "I don't know."

"You must love him so much," I said to her. I asked her more questions, trying to get her to explore her feelings, and I shared some stories with her concerning young mothers and adoptions. The most important thing, I knew, was that she be able to come to a decision on her own.

We talked for a while longer, looked at the adoptive families again, and talked about what the baby needed. Throughout the next couple of hours, I spent as much time as I could with her. The hospital counselor and the adoption agency representative came and spoke to her.

That afternoon Michelle decided she would give the baby up for adoption. I was there as she signed the papers with tears dripping down her cheeks. I know it was difficult to come to that decision, and I know she will grieve. I know she will physically heal from giving birth to her baby, but I also know she will forever carry the memory of her first child. I hope the memory will not always be painful. Even though I didn't do much for her, she had someone to talk with. I gave her permission to hurt, which gave her a little bit of reassurance and strength. That day I had a taste of the art of healing by using the simple act of caring.

RESPONDING IN ARGENTINA
by Rachel Contreras-Spencer (California, USA)

Once in a while everyone has one of those incredible experiences where one learns there is more to nursing than just the application of secular knowledge. I had the opportunity to experience such a moment in Argentina while working at a public maternity hospital. I learned to go beyond what I had learned in nursing school and discovered something that couldn't be taught. Seemingly forgotten, those babies in the "abandoned" section have taught me more than they'll ever know and will live on in my memory forever.

The hospital in Argentina was much like I had imagined it would be in a Third World country. It had six or seven floors, old tile, broken windows, no toilet paper or soap for the patients or doctors, about one nurse for every 40-plus mothers, and one nurse for every 16-plus intensive care infants. There were no private rooms to rejoice in when the newborn was delivered into this world. There were no private rooms where mothers could grieve when they experienced the loss of their child.

I had worked in the labor room and the postpartum unit, and on my last day, it was finally my turn to help in the NICU. I started feeding the babies and taking temperatures. When I was finished, a corner of the room caught my eye. I asked about the babies in this section and learned they were there because they were sick and/or abandoned.

It was known as the abandoned section because many of the parents of the sick babies couldn't afford to pay for medical costs. Parents were left with no alternative but to leave their child there in the hands of the government who would then pay to have them treated, if they didn't die first. The price parents paid was never seeing their child again.

Once they signed the paper, they weren't allowed to visit or care for their child.

The first baby I cared for was named Jose Ariel, and indeed he looked as though he had been forgotten. He had a heart abnormality and was lying in a little metal basket with a wet sheet, which reeked of emesis. He was not wearing any clothes, and his diaper was overflowing. I fed him, cleaned him up, and gave him one of the blankets and clothing articles I had brought from home. He loved the attention and was able to fall right to sleep.

I then moved on to Ivan who had hydrocephalus. He was 3 months old at the time and was scheduled to have a shunt placed within the next 2 days. The pressure that had built up was incredible. He had "sundowner's eyes" so severe that I could see only the whites of his eyes. His head weighed about twice as much as the rest of his body.

I went over, picked him up, and cradled him in my arms. I noticed the towel he'd been lying on was also wet, only it had no odor. I bathed him, clothed him, and held him. I had been watching his temperature and noticed there was a steady increase. It had gone up to 101.4 F. I spoke with some of the other student nurses who had been in there before. They told me that a day or two before some nurses had tried to relieve some of the pressure in Ivan's head by getting a little of the fluid out with a syringe and needle, but they neglected to place a bandage on his head. It soon occurred to me that the sheet was wet with cerebral spinal fluid.

I notified the pediatrician, and she said she'd be there when she finished making rounds. For me it seemed like an eternity. She confirmed that Ivan was leaking spinal fluid and most likely had an infection because his wound was left uncovered. Concerned about Ivan's upcoming surgery, I asked if it was likely they would go ahead and operate anyway. She replied it would be up to the surgeon.

When my arms grew tired of holding him, I tried to put him down, but he just cried uncontrollably. He loved being held, as if he had been starved for human contact. I had another student nurse hold him while I went to look for a bottle, which was no easy task. Returning about a half hour later, I held and fed him. He was ravenously hungry. I held him for hours and was able to feed him again before I left. I was the last to leave the unit, and my fellow students waited for me in the van. No one came in to hurry me along, because there was an unspoken under-standing.

While I held Ivan, I had plenty of time to think and reflect. I wondered what the future held for him. I watched as he lay complacently in my arms and wondered what kind of perfect spirit was inside his imperfect body.

I loved that I had the opportunity to help ease his great pain, if only for a day. The care I provided was not medical by definition; it was com-passion and love. I loved that I was able to help the helpless. I know that if I had not been there as a student giving service, Ivan wouldn't have been held and comforted. I would not have had the opportunity to show him there was someone who cared. I would have missed the lesson of a lifetime. It reaffirmed to me that I was supposed to be a nurse. I know of no greater profession wherein lies the opportunity to help heal others, both physically and spiritually.

My heart and mind go back to that place often and wonder if he ever made it to surgery and through recovery. I have since made a commit-ment to myself and to those I serve—that I will serve them as the Savior would serve them if He were here in my place. I want to convey to them my concern for their well being whether it is medical, emo-tional, or otherwise. I want them to know they are important.

NURTURING LIFE IN ALL ITS FORMS
by Angie Riches (Idaho, USA)

There is definitely an art to nursing, and I worked hard at my new job. I soon realized that labor and delivery was the place for me. I was able to be a part of the most amazing experience in most people's lives: I helped people celebrate and care for their new babies.

One experience I had not learned was the nursing art of dealing with death. I felt that maybe I chose labor and delivery because it was about life, not death. I knew that I would somehow have to learn to deal with this, and I struggled intellectually with how to give care to a family that was losing a baby.

I was still orienting when I took care of my first fetal demise. A beautiful young couple had been trying to have children for years. Just as they thought they had reached their goal, their baby's life ended before it had even begun. I cried that day, learning the pain that comes when there are no answers for what has happened. I could not celebrate the birth of this baby, nor could I fix what I so badly wanted to fix. I left that day with questions of how I should feel as a nurse in this situation.

Several months after this experience, I was working a regular night shift. In report, we were told there was a woman who came in because her membranes had ruptured. During admission, she explained to the nurse that her baby was special. He was going to be born with a disorder that was incompatible with life—meaning he would die. I deliberately did not take that patient; I did not feel that I could give her the care she deserved. Later that night, I heard this little boy had been born. I did not hear a cry come from the room, just silence. The father came out seeking someone who could help give his child a blessing before he died. We just happened to have a doctor who was a clergyman, and he came to help give the baby a blessing. Not long after that, the nurse came out and said that the baby had died. I swallowed the pit that had grown in my throat, and I said a little prayer for the family. It was about this time that the nurse asked if I could help her clean the room and change the linen.

At first, I was troubled, not sure I could handle seeing this disfigured family with their disfigured child. But, as I walked into the room, a great peace swept over me. The father was holding his son in his arms, and he had a smile on his face. He walked over to me and said, "Look at my beautiful son." As I looked at this perfectly formed child dressed in a white tuxedo, I felt a heavenly love for this child. This infant had come to earth for only a brief moment, but he touched everyone who came into contact with him. I smiled and knew this birth needed to be celebrated.

As I left that room, I realized what it was that I was feeling. It was the same thing I felt every time I saw a child born—it was joy. It is in these experiences, birth and death, that we get the closest to the veil of heaven that we will ever get. And at that moment, I knew what my role was—to nurture life in all its forms.

I did not have the answers for this family who had so many questions, but I did have the medical knowledge to help them understand what to do next. I could teach them how to take care of themselves and where to turn for help. Most importantly, though, I could tell this family the feelings I had as I entered their room and saw their beautiful child. I did not leave that day with a bitter feeling; I left with a peaceful feeling.

INCLUDING PATIENTS IN DECISION MAKING
by Jeffrey Ahsinger (Florida, USA)

This particular evening we had a patient expecting twins who had already had a prolonged hospital stay due to complications of pre-term labor. The time had finally come to deliver the twins, and she had been in the early stages of labor all day. She had been labeled by staff as difficult, as she had refused many of the interventions that are commonly used to establish labor. This evening, when the physician came in to assess cervical progression, he found the first twin had re-positioned itself causing a malpresentation, which meant that a vaginal delivery was no longer an option. After a lengthy explanation by the physician about why a cesarean section (C-section) was needed, the patient said she'd "had enough" and refused. Even after more explanation by the nurse caring for her, she still refused and was going to sign out against medical advice (AMA). I had been working on assistant nurse manager tasks during the day and had not been out on the unit. After hearing this story, I asked if I could go and give it a try. I was given the okay and armed with the AMA form and a cesarean section permit, so I headed toward the room.

I entered the room, identified myself, and said that I was here to remove her IV and had the papers she needed to sign. I was met with silence, squared shoulders, and a cold icy stare. I could tell by her body language that she was scared, confused, and angry. The natural defense—anger—was helping her remain in control. Who could blame her for her stance? All her hopes for a normal conclusion to this pregnancy had just been blown out of the water. Her significant other was seated quietly in the chair as she was gathering her belongings preparing to leave. I wasn't quite sure where to begin, so I just started talking, asking if she had any questions. But, she didn't respond. I asked her significant other if he had any. He shook his head "no." So again my mouth just started moving, and I spoke out loud about her prolonged stay due to pre-term labor and how difficult it must have been to hang in there for so long. That seemed to strike a chord. Her eyes started to fill with tears, and I told her it was okay and that I understood how frustrating it must feel for her that things just didn't go as planned. She sat down on the edge of the bed and cried hard. I thought we had made a connection, so I sat down next to the bed and gave her a minute to cry out her fears and frustrations. She finally talked to me, saying that this was not how she had planned the birth and that she felt we were making all of the choices for her. I realized then that she felt she had no control over what was happening, and I had to make her see that she really did.

I discussed the choices she had made already and the choices she still had to make. She had made the choice to give up a normal life to spend 6 weeks in the hospital, in bed, carrying these babies to term. She agreed and said that the planning of a normal delivery and healthy babies was what she thought about daily to help her get through. I told her that it must be incredibly sad and frustrating to plan for so long, only to have your dream shattered by yet one more complication. She agreed, and so did her significant other. I felt better now that all of us were in this conversation, and so I kept moving forward. I explained that she did still have control, and I wanted to tell her again what she could control. She said, "Okay, let's hear it," and gave a half smile. I told her that right now she had the ability to say yes to a C-section, get an epidural placed, and have a nice unrushed delivery. She would be awake and be able to see her children come into the world. She would go to recovery, with her epidural in place, and be alert enough to remember clearly the moment she first saw and held her children, knowing that the weeks in the hospital were not wasted time. She would also be pain free because of the epidural and not on medications that would cloud her memories. Her second choice would be signing out against medical advice, going home, and taking the chance that if her water broke and the first baby remained in a mal-presenting position, a medical emergency could occur. The infant's cord might prolapse, causing possible death to one or both of the babies due to compression of the baby's umbilical cord. Also, the driving time to the hospital and physician availability would factor into this picture for the outcome of these infants. Once here, she would be whisked off to the operating room (OR) for an emergency C-section where she would be put to sleep, with no one allowed to be with her, and she would wake up hurting and medicated, with clouded memories as a result. I told her she still had a third option, and it was that she could go home and hope labor would resume and all would go well.

Her significant other finally spoke up and voiced his desire to be in the OR when the babies were delivered. She was quiet, her body and demeanor more relaxed, and her tears had stopped. I told her that the choice was theirs, and I would leave, giving them the privacy to discuss what decision they would make. I also told them I had two forms on my clipboard, one would let her leave knowing it was against medical advice and the other was for a cesarean section, and she could sign whichever one she wanted. She smiled, thanked me for taking the time to listen to her and to discuss the situation with her without telling her what to do. She asked if I would be able to go with them to the OR. I told her that I would consider it a privilege. Forty-five minutes later, the proud father carried his two infant sons to the nursery after a successful C-section delivery.

I've learned that nurses often become task-oriented and empowered, thinking that we know what is right for the patient. This patient was not really given the chance to share her feelings. Neither had she or her significant other felt they were a part of the decision-making process. This caused unnecessary emotions like fear, frustration, and anger to surface. Unfortunately, she then got the rap as being "difficult"—all because she had the need and desire to feel like she had some decision-making authority over the path her life was taking. Once given the opportunity to express feelings and concerns, and to have someone listen, the couple was able to choose the best path to take for their family.

FACILITATING BONDING
by Sandra Blackington (Florida, USA)

The essence of care giving in the neonatal intensive care unit (NICU) goes so much beyond what is written in the orders or on my daily worksheet. Listening to cues given by the behavior of the infants creates a dialogue, which I integrate into my nursing care.

"She had a terrible night!" As shift-change report began, I quickly learned that one of the patients I would be caring for today, "Baby," had required increased ventilation, sedation, and frequent stabilization for dropping oxygen saturation levels throughout the previous night. "I had to call for a dose of Fentanyl, but even that hasn't seemed to help too much," reported her night nurse. I was also told she had been suctioned of copious secretions at both "touch times." Her abdominal girth had increased, she had not passed stool in 2 days, and her continuous feeding was stopped after she vomited. Today was the first time I had been assigned to the care of Baby in the 3 short weeks of her life in the NICU. While her history and current condition mirrored that of many other patients for whom I had cared in the past, I knew she would show me her unique individuality.

Baby's emergency cesarean section (C-section) birth to an 18-year-old primigravida at 28 weeks' gestation was complicated with maternal infection and asphyxia that required full code resuscitation. Weighing only 890 grams and not breathing on her own, she was intubated and placed on a ventilator where she remained since birth. Her course was complicated by respiratory distress syndrome (RDS), pneumonia, septicemia, and a feeding intolerance.

When report ended, I completed an assessment of both of my assigned patients, noting their general appearance, checking monitor readings, and infusing fluids. Baby was squirming away from the rolled blanket by her side and intermittently flexing her arms and legs. Her fists were tightly clenched. With this assessment and my report in hand, I knew that although Baby's next scheduled "touch time" was over an hour away, I planned giving her care much sooner. I wanted to determine the underlying cause of her instability and also saw opportunities to provide a more supportive environment. As I was reviewing the orders and medication sheets, Baby beckoned me to her bedside with an oximeter alarm. Baby, who had been pink when I checked only 10 minutes earlier, was now pale and dusky. She was expressing a voiceless cry, arching her back, with arms flailing rigidly. The oximeter reading had dropped to 65. Simultaneously I increased her oxygen, opened her isolette, and placed a hand over her chest, gently bringing her hands into mine. "What's wrong Baby?" I asked in a gentle voice. Her agitation gradually subsided and her color improved. With the momentary crisis behind us, I listened to her breath sounds to verify tube placement but found her aeration slightly diminished with crackles. I called the respiratory therapist to the bedside to ask if we could begin coordinating caregiving at this time. I suggested we should suction her first as it might help her tolerate the remainder of her care. After removing a large amount of secretions from her breathing tube, her breath sounds improved, and Baby appeared slightly more relaxed than before. I spoke quietly to Baby and noticed her eyes blink and her fingers splay in response to the noise of a closing isolette porthole. As I proceeded with my assessment, I was searching for both physical and behavioral cues. Her face and tiny eyelids looked puffy. Her brow was furrowed, and her arms and legs were extended as I gently cleaned her mouth. I noticed that she made no attempt to suck on the mouth swab or on the pacifier when it was offered. She seemed to respond to the sound of my voice as I spoke soothing words to her. She also clung to my finger when I placed it in her hand. I was pleased that she showed this self-comforting response. Although she had reached the corrected gestational age of 31 weeks, her current physical condition compromised her immaturely developed abilities to manage the stresses of her world. I helped her tolerate her care by pausing momentarily from time to time and placing my hands over her fragile body for containment. The remainder of her physical assessment revealed edema of the extremities; a full, soft abdomen with active bowel sounds; and no gastric residual. With an arterial line in one wrist and an intravenous line in the other arm, some of her usual opportunities to comfort herself by bringing her hands up to her face and mouth were inhibited. Having completed her care, I quickly formulated my plan for Baby's comfort and developmental support. I knew that appropriate non-pharmacological comfort measures would make a difference in her physiological responses. Gently, I lifted her into a "snuggle-up," a developmental positioning aid, and rolled her to one side. Flexing her arms and legs and bringing them to midline allowed her to place her hands in a comfortable position near her face. The head of the bed was slightly elevated, and she was given additional support with a flexible "Baby Bendy Bumper." These two fabric bands supported her fetal position.

The neonatologist arrived, and together we reviewed her current condition. I was comfortable with the decision not to have a narcotic ordered since Baby had shown a favorable response to some of the non-pharmacological interventions I provided. A diuretic and a glycerin suppository were added to her existing orders. I was anxious to administer the IV diuretic and decided to use floor stock rather than waiting for a pharmacy dose. I planned to administer the suppository at the next touch time.

Baby's mother called to ask about her condition. I had never met her mom, but I knew her visits had become less frequent and she had stopped expressing breast milk. She said she had a little cold. I reminded her that if she was not coughing and sneezing and did not have a fever, she could visit. She was silent. Then she said, "It probably doesn't matter if I visit." I asked, "What makes you feel that way?" She did not respond. I broke the silence by telling her she was a very special person in her baby's life. "You're her only mom. Yours is the voice that she heard echo in the womb. She needs to know your special touch." After a brief silence, mom said that she would see how she felt later. As I hung up the phone, I knew that we needed to help mom feel more a part of Baby's life.

A part of minimizing the stress of care given to babies is using an unhurried, relaxed, and gentle approach. Some might laugh when they hear my soft voice telling her what I am about to do, but somehow, it does make a difference. I offered her a pacifier, and she accepted it with a few sucks, then paused and brought her hand closer to her face. "Good girl," I whispered, knowing this non-nutritive sucking would make her feel calmer and help her digestive functioning. I spent a few extra minutes cradling her little body with my hand. I was able to wean her oxygen slightly.

Baby continued to improve throughout the afternoon. I continued to give close attention to other behavioral cues of discomfort, knowing they correlated with her physiological parameters.

A few days later, I met her mother. Telling Mom that it was about time for Baby's care, I suggested that we work together. She worked with me, and I complimented her and directed her attention to her baby's actions. I explained the benefits of supportive positioning, and she helped decide that we would support the baby in her "snuggle-up." Mom held Baby, and she seemed more relaxed and very engaged in what her baby was doing. Mom smiled and leaned closer, gazing at Baby's face. I stepped away from the bedside. I noticed she was speaking softly to her child. I knew this was another step in building the bonding relationship.

"One day at a time." These are frequent words I say to parents, and they are also the core of my caregiving. Every day I have an opportunity to enhance the healing process of my patients by using a holistic approach. The technology of neonatal care has dramatically increased survival rates. Nurses can and should lead the healthcare team in the integration of individualized, developmentally supportive, family-centered care.

Children. When you say that word you imagine playful, happy thoughts. You can see little girls swirling around in taffeta dresses; proud parents celebrating landmark birthdays; adolescents roller skating in the park, playing video games; and participating in their endless sporting events. We think of children like fountains of youth, enjoying eternal health and being problem-free. A toothless smile and bangs that are crooked—these are the faces of children.

Yet for many children, this is far from their reality. There are diseases that can't be cured, tumors not understood, and incredible journeys yet to take down the long hospital halls. The journey is where nurses make the difference. They give children a reason to be strong. They invent creative ways to divert pain. They make sure children are never left alone, even when the rest of the family has died in a car accident. They brighten, cheer, cajole, comfort. Nurses are there 24 hours a day, 7 days a week, day-in and day-out, during holidays, night shifts, and winter storms ... they are there for the sick kids in this world. They are also there for the families. It is priceless to the families when a nurse makes a 4-year-old more comfortable and eases her crying. The parents remember the nurses forever, and so do the children.

Some children have precious few resources. Continually, the nurses use their own money to buy toys, socks, CDs, and video games to help the child. Ask any nurse you know about what they have purchased for their patients, and you will learn the list is long. This is giving from the heart, a byproduct of a constant concern for others.

Are nurses the true heroes? Many nurses will say it is the children who are the heroes. How they fight their diseases and never complain is incredible. How they heroically try to comfort parents is unbelievable. One thing is for sure: When the patient needs the nurse and when the going gets tough, the nurse is always there—singing a lullaby, coloring a picture, teaching the parents, kissing the baby goodnight, and humming, "Everything's gonna be all right, rock a bye, rock a bye."

RECOGNIZING THE HERO IN SELF
by Maryann Godshall (Pennsylvania, USA)

I am writing this story to talk about those who are true heroes. They are not sports stars, movie stars, or even world leaders. The true heroes are children with cancer. I realized this fully the night I spent with a 17-year-old girl I will call "M." She was dying of acute lymphocytic leukemia (ALL). She had been diagnosed with leukemia when she was 11 years old. While other kids were playing, she was enduring chemotherapy. That alone is heroic. She had been doing well and was thought to be in remission, until recently when the unthinkable happened … she relapsed. Lately, we were giving her supportive care, transfusing blood products, and easing her pain with narcotics. She knew she was sick and dying but wanted to go home so she could go to the mall. She just wanted to go to the mall. What a simple request. Many people in the hospital made extraordinary efforts to get her home just once more. She was discharged on a Thursday evening and readmitted that Saturday in severe pain. M got to the mall twice in that short period. I was assigned to her that following Monday. As you might imagine, when I looked at my assignment and heard she was dying, I was saddened. I wasn't one of our unit's core group of chemotherapy nurses who knew her well. I had cared for M only a few times. I felt inadequate. I knew I would just try to do my best.

She was on a Dilaudid and Ativan drip, but she was still having pain. We gave her boluses of pentobarbital, which seemed to help. Her Ativan was discontinued and a pentobarbital drip was added to the Dilaudid for comfort measures. As I watched her struggle, I remembered the days when she walked the halls, talking to the staff and looking for things to do. I saw her parents and could not even imagine their pain. I have a 17-year-old and could not imagine saying goodbye. It seemed to me that all my caregiving actions seemed inadequate.

Even though she fought valiantly, she passed away just before 9 p.m. As I sat at the bedside with her parents and physician, I couldn't believe how hard she had fought. She was so brave for so long, and NEVER (as kids never do) complained or gave up. Her parents cried. I tried to be strong so I could help them. The pastor and chaplain on call were so very helpful. At that moment, I realized this was another gift of nursing: helping people to "die well." Not to die alone, but loved with family and friends by their side. I remembered a comment made by a pediatric oncology practitioner who said, "People ask me how I can do this, but how can I not?" I finally understood what she meant. What I thought was going to be a bad night turned into a beautiful experience I will cherish forever. How fortunate and privileged I was to be there when she took her last breath. My fellow staff members were so supportive.

On the drive home that night, I turned on the radio and heard Mariah Carey sing "Hero." Tears just rolled down my face. The words said:

"And when a hero comes along, with the strength to carry on,

When you cast your fears aside, you know you can survive.

And when you feel that hope is gone, look inside you and be strong,

And you'll finally see the truth, that a hero lies in YOU."

(Hero, Carey, 1993)

That is when I realized how much of a hero M was to have gone through what she did. She certainly was my hero. At the end, she even tried experimental treatments such as taking small amounts of arsenic to fight the cancer. She said if it didn't help her, it might help us learn more about cancer in order to save someone else. I couldn't believe those words were spoken by a 17-year-old.

But that is what kids do; they are unbelievably strong. Sometimes they try to be strong for their parents. If that isn't being a hero, I don't know what is.

Ironically the next song that came on was, "Everything's Gonna Be All Right, Rock-a-bye, Rock-a-bye." That was M. That's how she would like to be remembered. She used to wear headphones and listened to very up-beat music. Was that a message from her, I wondered? Weirdly enough, it brought me peace. I will always remember you M. We all will.

REALIZING THE PATIENT'S DREAM
by Tomomi Kameoka (Tokyo, Japan)

Miss Hiroko was a woman 40 years old. When she was a child, 9 or 10 years old, she experienced the first operation of her brain tumor. Her brain tumor was not malignant, but it returned many times after the operation. Whenever another new brain tumor returned, she had to experience the operations. She lost physical function gradually by aggression of the operations.

Miss Hiroko was hospitalized in a neurosurgery ward of a university hospital in order to be operated on. After the operation, some complications occurred, and she did not readily recover. She could not be discharged. We cared for her about 1 year, as her hospitalization was extensive. The conditions of Miss Hiroko were the following: She received a tracheostomy as respiratory care and received suctions of sputum by nurses every hour. She could communicate with others verbally but not smoothly because she used a speech cannula. Swallowing food was difficult for her, and she took food by using a nasal tube. She was not able to move either lower extremity or her right upper extremity by herself. She was not able to change position by herself. Therefore the nurses changed her position every 2 hours. Her right eye was lagophthalmos. Thus, the nurses gave her eye drops hourly in order to prevent drying and infection of her right eye. Her sweat nucleus had obstruction. Therefore she sweated severely. When the nurses visited her bedside, they wiped her body and changed her pajamas frequently.

Her condition hardly changed for a full year after the operation. One day the nurses had a conference about her nursing care. All nurses thought, "We provide sincere nursing care for Miss Hiroko every day. But her condition does not readily improve. Could we provide really sufficient care for her? How will she feel? What can we do for her? We have to think about it." After discussion, the nurses decided to ask her to confirm the perception of herself. A nurse asked her, "What is your first wish?" Each nurse imagined her answer. Some nurses imagined that her first wish was to eat food orally. Some nurses imagined that it was to leave the hospital.

The nurses were surprised to hear her answer. The first wish of Miss Hiroko was to write a card of thanks to persons who gave support to her. She was right-handed, but her right hand was paralyzed as a result of the brain tumor operation. As for the left hand, although it was not so smooth, she was able to move it a little. For example, she could use a wireless television remote controller with her left hand. One nurse recommended she use a word processor. She said, "I will challenge the word processor." Her mother bought a new word processor for her immediately. It was 10 years ago when few nurses could use a word processor in Japan. For most of the nurses at the neurosurgery ward, it was the first experience of using a word processor, but all nurses helped Miss Hiroko in order that she could master the word processor to write cards. Some nurses read the instruction manual of the word processor with Miss Hiroko. Other nurses tried to solve problems on the word processor with Miss Hiroko. After a month, she could finish writing a card beautifully. She expressed joy with a wonderful smile. And she thanked all the nurses very much. The nurses were very pleased that her wish came true. For the nurses, it was the best joy that her life had become rich.

ALLEVIATING PAIN
by Patti Lucarelli (New Jersey, USA)

Over the past few years, the compassionate treatment of patients' pain has finally come into its proper recognition and place in nursing care. This has always, though, been a respected component in my 25 years of pediatric nursing practice, with roots in my own childhood experience.

When I was 15 years old, I underwent emergency abdominal surgery for what eventually was severe cholecystitis and resultant cholecystectomy. Back then, a typical surgical procedure resulted in a week-long stay (can you imagine?), and the primary treatment for pain was meperidine intramuscularly. On my first day post-op, I was so miserable that no matter what I did I could not get comfortable, and certainly could not escape the burden of my post-op pain. Although sympathetic, the nurses could only offer the needle solution, which quite frankly made me sick to my stomach, and so I avoided asking for "the shot." How fortunate for me the mother of the young girl who was my roommate happened to be a nurse. Seeing my pain, she introduced herself and asked permission to help me. Of course I was willing to try anything, and with that, she briefly left the room, returning with several pillows tucked under her arms. She told me she was going to help position me so that I might be a bit more comfortable, and ever-so-gently she began rolling me while she placed the pillows strategically around my sore body. With each pillow in its proper place, she then gently rolled me on my side with pillows supporting my back, under my knee, and along my legs. With one final, gentle step, she delivered me into a spot where for the first time in the 24 post-surgery hours, I indeed had ah-h-h—NO PAIN!!! And what I can still recall in its finest detail and with incredible emotion (still) is that feeling of relief I experienced some 30 years ago!

I call it the "ah-h-h" phenomenon, and I have carried it with me to every patient for whom I have since been privileged to care. I see to it that each of my pediatric patients, whether undergoing treatments, immunizations, or suffering from the devastating effects of illness or disease, receives attention to and alleviation of his or her pain. There is no better satisfaction for me than to witness a child transform from painful misery to peaceful respite.

Likewise, I have been on a mission to help other healthcare professionals understand the importance of treating patients holistically and humanely, especially when it comes to pain management. I have spoken at many pain seminars and in-service training sessions, and I always invite the participants to journey back with me to my "ah-h-h" moments, as well as to remember their own "ah-h-h." I have witnessed how many of these nurses understand instantly, emphatically and empathetically, as they recall their own "ah-h-h" moments. This is because the power of relief is unforgettable. Whoever it was or whatever was done for them, once they experience that moment of relief, you know it's a powerful thing! When the "ah-h-h" becomes the goal (imagine putting that on the patient's care plan!), nursing care is compassionate, and treating pain no longer elusive.

"I was merely doing my job—taking care of a patient—to the best of my ability." This is a common statement among nurses. I am always amazed by it. Do nurses know how great they are? How they lighten the load in very touch-and-go situations. So often people say, "I could never do what you do as a nurse." Often, they are right. Only very compassionate, dedicated men and women can be true nurses. It is a profession for a select group of people who know what is good in life and what matters most. Their minds are creative and their strategies are incredibly effective. What nurses do is anything but ordinary—every day, they are truly making a difference.

LISTENING TO PATIENTS' STORIES
by Jane C. Hospador (Pennsylvania, USA)

Child abuse and neglect—ugly words conjuring up ugly visions of half-starved babies and toddlers with burned faces and unexplained bruises on their buttocks. There is no one who would want these things to happen to any child, and yet the national statistics regarding child abuse are staggering and continue to grow grimmer. Nurses often encounter abused children in busy emergency rooms, pediatricians' offices, or public health bureaus, or sometimes with their own friends or neighbors. Generally, abuse is not suspected until irreparable damage has been done.

In 1995, I was given the opportunity to become the coordinator and program manager for a new child abuse prevention program. Known as the PATH (Parent Advocate in The Home) program, it was created through the efforts of a concerned community and the support of a local philanthropist who cared deeply for children, particularly those disadvantaged children who had limited access to healthcare. I found myself carrying on the tradition of caring for children that had begun in 1919 by a community agency that provided a "milk bank" for new mothers who were unable to breast feed.

Our program model, in retrospect, was quite forward thinking. Its key components included:

1) A voluntary commitment on the part of the participating families.

2) Long-term, one-to-one intervention in the home setting.

3) Interventions that best met the specific needs of each family.

This was a time when current thinking on child abuse prevention supported group parenting educational classes outside the home and a structured curriculum with carefully defined objectives and outcome measurements. As I read up on the subject of child abuse prevention, I found that parenting programs could be started by just about anyone who cared about abuse. I also found out that nurses were rarely involved in these programs.

During the first few years, I struggled to explain our mission to community groups and potential financial supporters. Most wanted a "quick fix," viewing abuse only in the context of the physical damage done to children, and wanting me to provide a specific picture of what made a good parent. They had difficulty seeing a holistic picture in which the outside forces of poverty, lack of education, minimal health-care, and substandard housing, as well as the strengths of family pride and independence, resourcefulness, and daily coping strategies, all contributed to the child abuse and neglect environment.

My continued fight for my beliefs, even when it was hard to measure positive outcomes, comes from the story of "Laura." I had been with the program not quite 6 months when I met Laura. She had just had her first baby, and she was referred to us by a social worker because she had asked him for some support with parenting. As a child, Laura had been abused terribly, mostly by her mother. Laura showed incredible insight. She knew what abuse was all about, and she was terrified that she would repeat it on her daughter. Our home care mother-baby nurses who first intervened with Laura returned with alarming stories. My parent advocate and I scheduled a visit as soon as it was apparent that Laura was comfortable with our presence. This visit changed my life forever, as Laura became my teacher.

We entered a four-room home that reminded me of the company homes I had read about in novels set in Appalachia in the United States. It shared a common wall with a home that had been condemned. Bare wires were hanging from the ceiling. Wall studs revealed holes where rats traveled between homes. In places, the kitchen linoleum was worn down to the sub floor. In spite of all this, Laura kept her home almost spotless. She was determined to be a good hostess to her guests and had bought donut holes just before our arrival. She invited us for coffee and donuts. This was an invitation we could not refuse. We then sat down at a kitchen table that had a cage with several white mice as a "centerpiece." I decided not to say anything for the time being and just concentrate on the coffee and donuts. Fortunately, Laura was anxious to tell us all about her labor and delivery and how proud she was of her baby. I learned that Laura was a mother with great potential. Soon, the baby was making little stirring noises in her crib upstairs, and Laura couldn't wait to show her to us. Fortunately for me, I was now getting into more familiar nursing territory, and I quickly abandoned the remaining donuts and coffee.

As we entered the tiny little room, my attention was immediately drawn to the baby kicking and waving her arms in a spotless crib with bright crib bumpers. All the necessary baby items were carefully arranged beside her crib. It was only after I had taken all this in that I became aware of the baby's roommate, and quickly understood the need for the white mice in the kitchen. The roommate was a rather large (to me, a VERY large) boa constrictor in a glass aquarium-type cage. The wire mesh lid was held down by boxes of shot-gun shells! I have no idea what my face looked like as Laura rambled on with excitement about her new daughter. Thinking it best to keep my attention on the baby instead of the snake, I looked toward the baby only to notice a small bookshelf filled with expensive books on Hitler and the Third Reich. This was not quite as surprising as the snake, because our mother-baby nurses had already met the father who had told them he had 28 tattoos; one of them was a visible swastika. Back in my car, I pondered how to write my care plan.

My very brave parent advocate continued working with Laura for about 2-1/2 years. My written outcome measurements on Laura's completion of our PATH program do not tell the story you now know. Here is what my outcome measurements reported:

- The environment is safe and clean and appropriate for the child. (New home with yard, no boa constrictor, no shot-gun shells.)

- Appropriate-age toys are readily available.

- There is no evidence of domestic violence. (Laura is still living with the baby's father who travels as a truck driver and is away for long periods of time.)

- Client uses birth control methods to space children in her family. (Laura kept her promise that her children would be at least 2 years apart. She became pregnant when her daughter was about 2 years old.)

- Client shows ability to make positive decisions for herself and her family. (Through the efforts of the parent advocate, Laura opened a checking account and learned to balance her money. She also was able to buy a car in her name and pass her driving test. She has a part-time job in a mini-mart and tells us that she is being considered for promotion to a manager's position.)

- Child is in normal range for growth and development in both physical and cognitive ranges.

- Child is current with immunizations, and mother keeps her health appointments.

- There is no evidence of unexplained injury to the child. (Laura arranges safe, competent child care for her daughter during working hours.)

Is everything now perfect? Of course not. As hard as we tried, we could never persuade Laura to take her GED, even though she certainly could have passed it. But even with this apparent "failure," Laura has taught me something. Obtaining a GED is not only an academic accomplishment, but it is the start of a redefinition of the whole person. Laura could never quite take that step that redefined her as a totally competent person who could take on responsibilities of greater magnitude. I remember this when I get frustrated at one of our mothers who could have a better life if only she would obtain her GED.

I last spoke with Laura at her mother's funeral service. Laura had begged us to come, saying we were the most important people to her. My parent advocate and I were saddened by the continued pathologic relationship Laura had with her mother, and we could barely stand the suffering she was now undergoing with her mother's death. Laura echoes the cry of so many adults who were abused as children. "She may not have been the best mother, but she was the only mother I had." Did I make a difference? As I look at her effervescent toddler, who quickly runs with arms wide open to my parent advocate, I see a beautiful, eager, trusting child who embraces life and those around her. As I get in my car, I can only imagine this child as an adult saying, "I had a great mother. I want to be like her when I have children." She is too young to remember the nurses who came and visited her for her first 2 years of her life, but maybe some day Laura will tell her about us. And as I continue on, family by family, Laura helps me explain our mission and how we prevent child abuse and neglect by listening to the stories and lessons our families tell us.

LEARNING A LESSON
by Jackie Whiting (Florida, USA)

As I walked into Ellen's room, I had no warning that this would be a very painful visit for me—a visit, in fact, that was haunted by an old ghost. My job as an advanced practice nurse in mental health requires frequent therapy sessions with patients. These are often difficult with challenging patients, and Ellen certainly was a challenging patient.

Ellen was involuntarily admitted. Her mother was concerned that she wasn't "making sense" and brought her to the emergency room (ER). She had not been eating or sleeping well and had been isolating herself from family and friends. She was an 18-year-old college freshman who had been valedictorian of her prestigious high school. She had no previous psychiatric history.

I remember reviewing possible pertinent factors to explore: Was there a family history of mental illness or substance abuse? Had the patient recently been involved in a stressful relationship? The admission assessment was limited due to the patient's confused state. The mother was not present after the initial ER assessment and had not talked to the mental health evaluators. That seemed unusual, but not enough to raise a warning flag. Her laboratory work showed anemia, dehydration, and other results in the low-normal range, such as the potassium level. You will often see this in a paranoid patient who has stopped eating. I wondered if this was a first schizophrenic break. Ellen's mother reported to the ER staff that her daughter had been dieting and had lost about 10 pounds since starting college in August. Well, a 10-pound weight loss in 4 months wasn't excessive. Ellen was 5 ft. 6 in. tall and weighed 108 pounds.

Armed with that limited knowledge, I entered Ellen's room. I saw a young girl who looked more like 13 than 18, dressed in baggy pants and a sweatshirt. She looked up as I entered the room, but she showed no emotion. The lights had been turned off and the blinds had been drawn. Even in this dim atmosphere, I could see that her limp hair lacked luster. Ellen had not taken any effort with her appearance and seemed to shrink into her clothes. As I approached her, I noticed the sharp bone structure visible beneath tightly drawn skin. "Oh my God," I thought. "This is Jenny all over again."

Do you have a patient who haunts you? One you always remember with questions like: "Did I miss something?" "Could I have done something differently?" Well, that's my Jenny. I met Jenny during my first month on the psychiatric unit. She was a young-looking 18-year-old who was very attractive, with the biggest brown eyes I'd ever seen. Her 5 ft. 3 in. height and her strict upbringing gave her an air of innocence that was almost childlike. Her parents had divorced 8 years earlier, and her father had been awarded custody. Jenny hadn't seen her mom in 7 years and had only received the occasional postcard from her during that time. Her mom was in and out of hospitals and psychiatric treatment programs. Her father was a prominent dentist who prided himself on the educational achievements of his only child. She had graduated from high school 1 1/2 years early and had immediately started her challenging college courses. Her father discouraged her association with her former classmates because he believed they were immature and a bad influence. Jenny was effectively isolated from her peers, with no one to talk to about the insecurity she was experiencing in college.

She and her father set goals for her that would have Jenny graduating from college by the age of 20. She planned to start medical school immediately after that. Jenny had always been a compliant child and eager to please her father. He said in one session with counselors, "I never thought she would turn out to be crazy like her mother." Jenny had glared at him, crossed her arms, and refused to participate any more that day. "I don't know what's wrong with everybody. Why are you keeping me in the hospital? There's nothing wrong with me!" She cried again and again. At that time she weighed 80 pounds; was consuming no more than 300 calories a day; and had abnormal labs, chronic constipation, and an abnormal EKG. When staff talked to her about the need to eat, she angrily demanded, "Why are you trying to control me? Do you want me to stay fat so no one will ever talk to me?" It is characteristic of persons with anorexia to deny they have an illness. They also frequently refuse to cooperate with treatment.

Doctors, dietitians, and psychiatrists all pleaded, threatened, and cajoled her in their efforts to get her to eat more. Nursing staff had strict orders to have her sit at the desk for meals, stay at the desk for one-half hour afterward, obtain daily weight reports, and limit her physical activity. She would cut her meat into miniscule bites and hide the pieces under her potatoes. She would fill her pockets with uneaten food in efforts to fool us. Her best trick was to conceal rocks in her robe pockets to add precious ounces to her daily weights. She would also drink copious amounts of water for a similar effect. Nothing we did seemed to make a difference.

I was Jenny's appointed nurse for more than a month. We began to build rapport. She would ask me about the high school activities of my children and tell me her dreams of someday being rich and famous and driving a red Corvette. "My dad won't let me get my driver's license until I maintain a 4.0 grade-point average for four semesters," she shared. "I would love to get in a car and just drive across the United States. No worries, and no pressures of tests, just to be totally free!"

Little by little her weight began to increase. Her eyes became brighter, and her smile more frequent. She would tease me, saying things like, "I'll specialize in psychiatry, and I'll come back and bug you all with orders." She began to share her feelings of abandonment by her mother, and she talked about her loneliness and her lack of friends or boyfriends. She began testing her flirting abilities with the male staff. I was so happy that I had been a contributor to her success.

The proud day finally arrived when Jenny was discharged. "I want to thank you for all you did," she said. "I'll remember you all my life." She was smiling and had gained 13 pounds. I wished she could have stayed a little longer; I had an uneasy feeling that just wouldn't disappear. The family sessions with her father were still difficult, and there was no resolution to key issues.

Less than 2 weeks later, we heard the news that Jenny had left home and her father couldn't find her. I remember wondering what could have happened. Was she just fooling us? This was not a sophisticated hospital, but we had used appropriate interventions. I also began to feel anger. I had worked so hard with Jenny.

Jenny never did return. She was found dead in a run-down apartment building in a nearby urban area. She starved herself to death and was not found for several days. "What a waste of a young life with so much promise!" I thought. I also felt guilty. I had missed so many hints that Jenny was back into people-pleasing, faking her wellness to gain discharge. I hadn't been forceful in stating my concerns.

When I faced Ellen, old thoughts and feelings overwhelmed me. "I'll do everything right this time; I won't be fooled again." Ellen didn't make her recovery any easier than Jenny had. She challenged the expertise of all the staff throughout her stay. This time we knew more about this terrible disease of anorexia. We recognized the manipulation, we treated her with new antipsychotic drugs, and we reached stabilization with Ellen. We also had frequent team conferences, both with and without Ellen, and we invited her to join the creative planning of her treatment. Our goals were to put her in control of her recovery.

Ellen's story had a happy ending. She has been in recovery for several years, and she maintains her ideal weight. There are still occasional difficulties with her mother, but nothing that Ellen can't handle. Interestingly enough, Ellen has chosen to be a dietitian.

When I was Jenny's nurse, I was so caught up in the helper role. With further education and many years of experience, I relearned that the patient's needs come first. I didn't try to mother Ellen. I really listened to her. I didn't suggest solutions; but was there to help her explore her own solutions.

Two-thirds of the patients with anorexia recover fully with prolonged aftercare, but there are still anorexia victims who die. Death can result for those who do not continue in active therapy or who have families who cannot stay the course of treatment.

I will remember Jenny for the rest of my life. I am grateful for the lessons she taught me. I don't want to look back in pain anymore. Jenny is free. I choose to believe there is a heaven, and I picture Jenny driving around in that bright red Corvette, free from the ghosts that haunted her. I could be a better nurse for Ellen because of the lessons I learned with Jenny.

Stories are accounts of life moments. They are carved into the minds of nurses. They are part of their personal past, shared with us to feel, touch, and breathe. The work of nurses devoted to women and children is nursing at its best. Shining stars, these men and women have gifts to be admired and cherished—hearts as big as the ocean, brainpower that can move mountains, and personalities as gentle as a cool breeze on a summer night. Nurses of women, children, and their families are blessed spiritually, academically, and physically to nurse this special population.

REFERENCES

Carey, Mariah. (1993). Hero. On Music box [CD]. Los Angeles, CA: The Island Def Jam Music Group/Universal Music.

Grubesic, R., & Selwyn, B.J. (2003). Vitamin A supplementation and health outcomes for children in Nepal. *Journal of Nursing Scholarship*, 35(1), 15-20.

Hartley, L. (2002). Examination of primary care characteristics in a community based clinic. *Journal of Nursing Scholarship*, 34(4), 377-382.

Pillitteri, A. (1999). Maternal and child nursing. Care of the childbearing and childrearing family (Third edition). Philadelphia: Lippincott.

Santacroce, S.J. (2003). Parental uncertainty and posttraumatic stress in serious childhood illness. *Journal of Nursing Scholarship*, 35(1), 45-51.

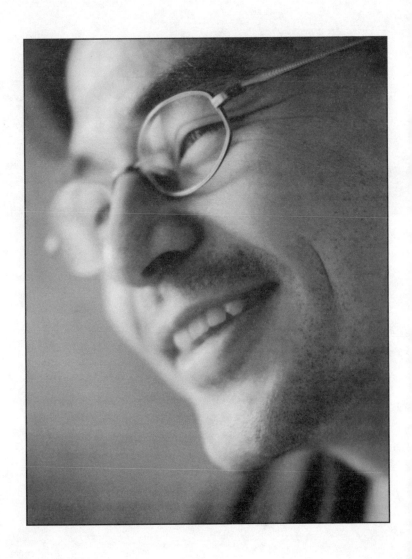

CHAPTER 4

Cultural Competence: Working Within Religious and Ethnic Frameworks

Religion and spirituality are central for patients experiencing a crisis. The spiritual beliefs and needs of patients are tremendously diverse. Patients representing many religious denominations pass through the halls of healthcare facilities every day. Respect for all religious faiths and practices are a priority goal. Nurses appreciate the need for Scripture reading, prayer, and other expressions of faith in a god as patients often use prayer to cope in times of illness. Similarly, they meet with spiritual leaders during the course of a patient's illness. During births, illnesses, and deaths, the nurse is often present for the spiritual experiences of the patient and his or her family.

Spiritual distress can occur when individuals are disconnected from their religious ties or cultures. Patients will express these concerns to the nurse. If solutions are possible, they should be implemented early. Nurses write goals and specific plans of care that include the spiritual needs of patients. These may include assessing beliefs and preferences, informing patients of spiritual resources, and creating an environment that is conducive to free expression. Other areas the nurse facilitates include identifying support systems, listening to patients and families, and providing privacy for quiet meditation (Swearingen & Ross, 1999).

Sometimes, spiritual conflicts can greatly affect one's health status. Jehovah's Witnesses cannot accept blood products and the administration of blood during surgery (Spector, 2004, pp. 113-115). Abortion, refusal of nutrition, and suicide are also major areas of conflict that confront nurses. Moral and ethical dilemmas challenge the nurse's own belief system. Knowledge of these potential conflicts and of cross-cultural healing traditions is essential to nurses. Nurses have a history of recognizing and affirming religious practices for those in their care (Weaver, Flannelly, & Flannelly, 2001). For example, in some cultures, candles are used after death to light the way for the soul of the deceased. In China, jade stones are placed in the orifices of the deceased to prevent evil spirits from affecting the body. Irish Catholics pray aloud using a rosary as a stepping-stone to the Virgin Mary (Spector, 2004, pp.126-7, 152). Diverse cultural practices are revered and facilitated in many nursing settings: in hospitals, home care, hospices, and long-term care, to name a few.

Nurses see patients and families fulfilled and comforted by their practices. They are actively involved with patients, saying a rosary or reading a prayer card. It is not uncommon for the nurse to be the only person there in the home or at the hospital bedside when the patient dies. It is the nurse who seeks the spiritual link, as the patient is ready to pass on to the next life. Nurses are comfortable soothing a patient and understanding the patient with spiritual needs. Most nurses are at ease using prayer to connect with patients. The nurse-patient relationship is sacred, holy, consecrated. The presence of a god and the nurturing of a strong religious faith are evident in the narratives that follow.

NONDENOMINATIONAL NURSING
by Charles Kemp (Texas, USA)

During a clinic session at Midpark Place (an early clinic site in the Kurdish community), I fell into conversation with an elderly man who had brought a Russian Jew to the clinic to pick up medications. I noted the elderly man had a faded series of numbers tattooed on the inside of his arm, horrifying proof he had been in a Nazi concentration camp. In that same room at that same time, there were Baylor students (mostly Baptist), Catholic volunteers, Kurds (mostly Muslim), an Armenian family (history shows that Kurds participated in the attempts to exterminate the Christian Armenians 1894-1915), and a Buddhist caseworker. Moments like this help me remember the beauty and power of this work.

STEPPING OUT OF THE COMFORT ZONE
by Marlene Cesar (Florida, USA)

In 2000, I was working as a clinical nurse and coordinator of the Hemophilia Program in the Department of Pediatrics at a Florida hospital. There were 164 patients in the program at that time, aged 0 to 17 years. In this country, most diagnoses for hemophilia are made in infancy, which reduces the risk of complications over the long term. My job was to visit the patients every Thursday, with the hematologist, the orthopedist, and the clinical social worker. Our practice model was a holistic one.

My job was routine until May 2000, when I received an e-mail, followed by a phone call from a wonderful activist and mother ("Jean," name changed) of a son with hemophilia, who was a prominent and wealthy person in our community. Thus began one of the most challenging, professional, and physical journeys I have ever undertaken!

The request was urgent; we had to go to Mayreau Island in the southern-most part of the West Indies, one of the many islands that make up St. Vincent and the Grenadines. On Mayreau Island, we met Mary, a desperate mother of two boys, Kishroy, age 6, and Kishron, 4, both diagnosed with hemophilia. Mary reached out for help from a remote but beautiful island, where the nearest medical facility was a day's travel by ferry boat and plane to St. Vincent.

Mayreau is a poor community, accessible only by boat. It has no available healthcare systems, with the days measured by the weekly delivery of supplies from the mainland. Mayreau was something less than paradise for this family. Indeed, it was a prison, especially for the boys. And hemophilia was their warden, with no healthcare, no Factor VIII for infusion, no doctors, and no easy way out.

The two boys had been in pain for years, with swollen legs in casts—dangerous treatment when there is uncontrolled bleeding. Resources were very limited; fresh frozen plasma, an obsolete method of treatment, was all the doctors could offer to the boys whenever Mary took them to St. Vincent. The boys were unable to play or run because of constant pain.

I had to make up my mind to participate in the escape plan initiated by a desperate mother and her amazing efforts that demonstrated a mother's love that knew no bounds. The university I worked for had no budget for this type of service, and my decision to help was a personal one. I secured the authorization of the medical director of the Hemophilia Program to take some days off to accomplish my noble rescue mission. I was only allowed to take personal days without pay. However, I was granted permission to use all available teaching materials such as simulated arms, IV packs, infusion information and equipment, along with syringes and other miscellaneous medical equipment used in the clinic for our hemophilia patients. I obtained a year's supply of Factor VIII for the boys' use. The cost of my trip was sponsored by Jean, who provided funding for teaching and caring for patients with hemophilia worldwide.

Although the trip was paid for, the travel was by a difficult and circuitous fashion, requiring a flight from Miami to Puerto Rico and then to Antigua, followed by a flight to St. Vincent and then on to Union Island. From Union Island, a speedboat carried passengers on to Mayreau, a small mountainous island. After docking, a pick-up truck was used to take me around the island.

My dilemma? I have a fear of flying, and the smaller the plane, the greater the fear! However, I realized that the importance of the mission I was about to take on was greater than my fear. I needed to be there. I was the only one who could teach Mary and the available medical personnel what was necessary to ease Kishroy and Kishron's pain and to prolong their lives. I was scared but determined to go, and even more determined to succeed.

Although I had never met Jean, we were to meet in Antigua. At the San Juan airport, I was quite concerned the travel arrangements might fall through and I would have to go on this "daring adventure" alone. I began to pray and took out my rosary beads on the plane to Antigua. I was approached by another traveler on the plane because she saw me "fingering my rosary beads" during the flight. She stated later that because it was obvious I had a great fear of flying, she felt I must have been one of the most committed people she had ever met.

When we finally landed, the time to start on our rescue mission had arrived. As soon as we unpacked and got situated, we went straight to meet with Mary and the boys. I was particularly touched by the plea of this mother who had suffered with her boys for years.

Mary said she received a book, Raising a Child with Hemophilia written by Jean, from a tourist visiting Mayreau. This was her "tremplin" (bridge) to reach out for help, and she had already started reading the book and was faithfully waiting for help. Soon we arrived at her humble home. She was ready to learn how to infuse. I quickly assessed Kishroy and Kishron who had already lost a lot of function with their knees affected by long periods of bleeding (hemarthrosis). I gathered some subjective data from the mother, and I understood quickly that hemophilia was considered to be a curse on a family as evidenced by their cultural beliefs. "My family wanted to know what I had done to bring this to our family," she told me sadly. As an islander myself, I could relate to her feelings. Even though I have espoused Madeleine Leininger's theoretical concepts on congruent cultural care, I was aware of the strength of the cultural belief systems in the Caribbean area.

I was concerned I would not have enough time to teach the mother, and I had a greater concern that there was no accessible medical support in case the boys developed an allergy to the Recombinant Factor VIII. The teaching experience was gigantic, in more ways than one, as the mother was not an educated person but was determined to succeed. Mary was ready to learn and eager to be able to infuse her children at home to decrease the burden of traveling to St. Vincent. After the first 2 hours of teaching, the mother was able to demonstrate IV insertion and infusion delivery.

Over the next few hours, I gave the mother information that would have taken months to impart to a family in the United States because of access. This type of teaching varies in the United States as the child matures, or as changes in treatment occur. On Mayreau, I had only one opportunity, and it had to count. Lives were at stake. I reviewed educational materials and information, such as joint exercises, pain management, treating bleeding episodes, monitoring for allergic responses, and most importantly, the logging of infusions and documenting amounts, times, and reason for administration of Factor VIII.

Normally, the parents bring a child's log to the hemophilia center. This mother had to communicate her treatment protocols long-distance to the closest medical personnel, on nearby Union Island, a 45-minute and $50 (US) speedboat trip away. To assist her follow-up, Mary suggested we needed to go there the following day to provide an in-service to the medical personnel on that island. Great! A speedboat ride again the following day, with the same boat captain, a cocky 14-year-old with a "need for speed." But first, we had to finish out our day on Mayreau, solving almost insurmountable problems, such as, where to store the Factor VIII, which has to be refrigerated. The family had no electricity. It was finally decided the infusion products would be stored underneath the parents' bed, which was the coolest place in the house, in a special cooler normally used for transporting perishable medical items.

We closed out the long day with a dinner celebration with the family as the island grew darker with the setting sun. The final toast was for the mother for her positive attitude, perseverance, and determination. It was her birthday. She had just turned 30.

The next day we were off to Union Island on the speedboat, accompanied by Mary, where we met the local doctor and three registered nurses. The clinic was not open that day because it was Sunday. Everyone participated in the in-service about hemophilia and the treatment protocols for this dread disease. Along with the teaching information and materials, we left contact numbers in Miami for information and help in case of emergencies.

We also left a supply of Factor VIII concentrate in the refrigerator at the clinic as the mother's backup supply. By four o'clock that afternoon, we said our farewells and were on our way to St. Vincent by plane, and on our way back to Miami early the next morning! This was only a 2-day trip, but with a profound and life altering impact on all involved. I was glad I had made this trip. This family is proof that it's not only education and wealth that can bring happiness. These people had so little and yet they were happy. Mary was still able to laugh and take on life's challenges. It was a big achievement and quite meaningful for me to be able to teach this mother how to care for her children in a manner that will improve their life expectancy.

Mary is still caring for Kishroy and Kishron and receiving Factor VIII via express delivery services. She has eliminated her treatment trips to St. Vincent because she is managing the infusions at home. Through Jean's efforts, Mary received a grant to start her own T-shirt business and was recently able to buy a refrigerator—now that electricity has been introduced to the island. I was asked to return to the island for a follow-up visit, and I am strongly considering it, even if I have to fly. I consider this experience a paradigm of all my clinical experiences.

I believe it is my duty to share my talents with my brothers and sisters, wherever they may be. As a nurse, I must help and share, laugh and suffer with my patients. A human being is not complete unless he or she can share with others. Giving of oneself is the greatest gift.

Three women came together from vastly different backgrounds on a remote island for one very special purpose. Martha Rogers, nurse theorist, believed nursing occurs wherever people are, even on remote islands. Nurses have to be willing to step out of their comfort zones, even when they are afraid to fly.

LISTENING TO THE WHISPERINGS OF THE SPIRIT

by Judy Malzahn Ellsworth (*The Healer's Art*, p.76)

Working in the operating room (OR) is an opportunity for never having a dull moment. Our hospital is just blocks off the western end of the Washington, D.C., Beltway. Each day brought new challenges, which meant we had to be ready for anything.

I was working as the assistant head nurse in charge of the OR from 4:00 p.m. until midnight 5 days a week. One Sunday afternoon I got a call from the delivery room telling me they had a very serious situation. A mother who had just delivered was hemorrhaging, and they were unable to control it—did we have an operating room available? We had four rooms running, and that was the maximum we could run that afternoon. I told them I would call them right back. I talked with someone in the anesthesia department, and we decided I could scrub for the case. We would pull a circulator from a case that would be finishing within the hour to circulate for me if delivery would send an RN down to circulate in the "easy" room. Arrangements were made with the critical care supervisor to watch the OR desk, and the go-ahead was given for the case to proceed.

I rushed to scrub and set up the room. While I was busy, the doctors brought the anesthetized patient into the room, prepped her for abdominal surgery. I put all the drapes on a table and told the doctors they were on their own, as I was still opening instruments and setting up. By the time I completed these tasks, I had gowned and gloved a doctor and two residents, and the patient was fully draped and ready to go.

The case was a serious one. This was in the days before the "Bovie," so we had to clamp and tie each bleeder. Every time a bleeder was clamped, the clamp acted as though it was like a hot knife going through butter. We tried to use a needle and tie off the bleeders. This didn't work any better. We packed her abdomen and waited to see if the bleeders would clot off. This was not successful. The situation was getting desperate.

I was feeling heartsick at our seemingly helpless situation. I knew this particular physician needed help. I felt like the patient was my sister, and I could feel the tears beginning to sting my eyes. I was the charge nurse, and I was the scrub nurse for the case and unable to call for help. While we were waiting to see if packing the abdomen was going to be successful, I turned to my back table; closed my eyes; and pleaded, Heavenly Father, please send someone quickly! This new mother needed more help than this surgeon was able to give her.

About 10 minutes later, the door to the operating room opened slightly and the chief of OB/gyn looked inside. He said he'd been out on a Sunday drive with his boys, and he felt like he needed to stop in at the hospital to see how everything was going. The doctor who was operating explained the situation, but he said he thought he had everything under control. The chief asked the doctor if he could use another hand, to which he said, "No!" I was shocked, and I looked at the chief and said, "I have an extra gown here, what size gloves do you wear?" (He later told me the look in my eyes told him he'd better start scrubbing immediately!)

We worked for 3 more hours, with the chief eventually taking over the case. The patient was saved, and I said several prayers of thanksgiving while we were working.

When the patient was taken to the post anesthesia care unit (PACU), I realized the doctors and circulating nurse had forgotten to take the patient's chart with them. I picked up the chart and started to take it to PACU when I read the name of the patient. Imagine my shock when I realized my impressions of the patient being my sister were very close. She had been my friend when we both lived in Seattle, Washington, several years before! Neither knew that the other was also living in the Washington, D.C., area.

I called up to the delivery room and asked if her husband could come down to the recovery room. I then made arrangements to allow for him to give her a spiritual blessing. I am grateful I was taught to listen to spiritual whisperings and act accordingly.

MEETING PATIENT NEEDS IN CUBA
by Kathryn Gaylord (Washington, USA)

I was deployed to Operation Joint Endeavor in 1994. This was a task force set up to process Cuban and Haitian refugees on the U.S. Naval Base at Guantanamo Bay, Cuba. My role was officer in charge (OIC) of a psychiatric inpatient unit. The unit was first established in a tent but was quickly moved to a solid facility following our first suicide attempt by hanging via tent ropes.

There are many poignant stories about events that occurred during my 6-month deployment, but this one was truly a miracle. Two of my patients, Julio and Marie, each lost their only sons in an attempted refugee boat trip to the United States. In their quest for a new life for themselves and their families, each lost their child and much of their hope. Interestingly, these sons shared the same name, Aaron. Each of these parents experienced deep depressions and attempted suicide many times. They were on a continuous 1:1 watch for several months. They both believed that their lives were now useless and hopeless.

Upon hearing that Julio and Marie were both Catholic, I arranged for a special mass to be held at the psychiatric unit. The intent of the service was for healing. The priest, a Cuban-American, said the mass in Spanish and English. He surprised us by setting up an altar with a picture of the Blessed Mother. He also brought the adult and children's choirs that had been formed in the camps. The sound of the children singing brought tears to everyone. The entire unit attended the service, regardless of religious affiliation. What I observed was surely the presence of God on earth. Following the service, neither Julio nor Marie attempted suicide again. They were finally able to share their sons' lives and were both able to move forward in therapy. Eventually Julio and Marie made their way to the United States.

RECOGNIZING AN ASSUMPTION
by Charles Kemp (Texas, USA)

I was seeing a 50-year-old woman with diabetes and an infected toe, which frequently occur together—horribly in some cases. Somewhere during the exam I realized she worked at a major hospital. I was irritated. We are a small, overloaded mission clinic, serving people who have nowhere else to turn, and of course, this woman had insurance. I told her we would take care of her infected toe and tide her over with oral hypoglycemics. I also told her she should use her insurance and see a private doctor or go to the hospital clinic. While I was getting her medications, she told Lupe (our promotora) that she worked for a temp service and did not have insurance. Lupe told me when I came back into the exam room. I felt small, so much for my cheap irritation. I asked the woman to come back in the following week first thing in the morning, fasting, so we could get a better picture of her blood glucose. She then told us she worked a split shift—6-10 a.m. and 4-8 p.m. Have you ever worked a split shift? It is really hard—you're never really off. So this is the life our patients lead—very, very hard, out of medications half of the time, putting up with irritated clinic people. When she returned 3 weeks later (no diabetes meds for the last 2 weeks), she told Lupe she actually did have insurance but did not know how to use it. This also is the life many lead, paying (top dollar, I might add) for something they cannot use. She is scheduled to return next week for a blood glucose check and help from our social worker to be able to use her insurance.

SHARING SPIRITUALITY,
by Marty Downey (Idaho, USA)

Three years ago I received a phone call from a nurse colleague and friend that changed my life. My friend, Jill, is a case manager for individuals and families living with congestive heart failure (CHF) in our community. She is supported in this role by a local regional medical center. Jill and I met through our mutual interest in critical care nursing and our participation in the local chapter of the American Association of Critical-Care Nurses. We took the certification examination together and extended our education together in a Master of Science in nursing program. Jill was also aware of my interest in holistic nursing and massage therapy, which is why she contacted me regarding one of her patients.

Jill had been assigned to manage the care of an 80-year-old woman named Susan with CHF who had a long history of signs and symptoms of heart failure. Susan's health was improving due to Jill's weekly visits and counseling. One area that was difficult for Jill to manage was Susan's chronic hip pain. Jill called to ask if massage therapy might help ease

Susan's pain. I could tell from Jill's description of Susan that this patient held a special place in Jill's heart. I explained to Jill I would arrange to visit Susan to determine whether I could be of any service to her.

My first contact with Susan was by phone call to set up an appointment. At this time, I also spoke to her husband, Vic, and it was evident he was part of Susan's healthcare. Vic and Susan welcomed me into their condominium a few days later. They delighted in showing me their home and the many flowers they nurtured around the condominium, and in sharing the joy they received from viewing several pairs of birds outside their patio doors. Both husband and wife were well informed about their healthcare decisions. Although I thought I was there to assess Susan's health needs, I soon found they were also assessing me. They asked questions that gave me a sense they would only accept the best of care. I was immediately aware of the deep passion and spirituality that were the sustaining forces in their home. After determining I was a knowledgeable nurse, Susan asked if I was a Christian. I answered yes, and I soon came to understand the importance of that affirmation in our relationship with one another over the years.

At the conclusion of the first visit, we agreed to try some massage therapy and body movement instructions to help Susan continue to stay active. Her long-standing scoliosis was a factor in her hip pain. The most I could do was to relax her muscles, which would enhance her comfort level. I allowed Susan and Vic to determine whether they wanted to continue the therapy each time I visited, and soon I was seeing Susan on a weekly basis. Susan seemed to respond well to the massages and the bits of education related to body movement. We discussed everything from family to flowers. She especially enjoyed the company and the sense of spirituality that we shared. When Jill and I compared notes, it was evident Susan was influential in Jill's spiritual life as well.

Between Jill's weekly check-ups, Susan's healthcare visits, and my massages, Susan managed to remain active the first 6 months. There were only two distinct setbacks, one was an episode in their winter retreat where she received a pacemaker and the other was for hyponatremia that set Susan in the hospital for a week. After this, Susan and Vic moved into a retirement center. Vic was vigilant about the care he gave to Susan. He made certain that Susan took the medications exactly as prescribed. He kept track of her weight and blood pressure. He made certain all of her appointments were kept. Vic was a genius at finding assistive devices to enhance Susan's activities, and he kept her spirits up with prayer and love. He even managed to place a special attachment in their bedroom window that allowed Susan to view the local birds! He also brought her flowers as often as possible.

Although the team effort to sustain Susan's health was strong, her strength slowly declined. Each week I could see a change in her self-care abilities. Some weeks, as I massaged, I would note an increase in her ankle and foot edema that would improve the next week due to Jill's intervention and medications. Throughout all of this care, Susan never complained, and she remained steadfast in her faith. We spoke often about our religions, the differences and the commonalities. She gave thanks each time I visited and declared me a blessing. Susan touched me deeply, and it was clear that Susan was the real blessing.

One week, I decided that my exposure to a cold/flu virus might be detrimental to Susan, so I called and reluctantly informed Vic that I would skip that week and see Susan the next. Unfortunately, there would not be another week for me to visit. Jill left a message on my work phone that Susan was experiencing dyspnea, worse than she had ever experienced previously and asked that I call her. By the time I received the message, Jill had spent a full day and night at Susan's bedside, along with Vic, family members, and their pastor. Jill described Susan's last moments to me, sharing her feeling of being honored at being at Susan's side as she transitioned into the next life. We cried together at the loss of our special friend. We both believe Susan had been a shining light for us and that there would be an incredible void in our lives now.

At her funeral, Vic and family friends described Susan in ways that brought more awareness to Jill and me. It was a celebration of a spirited woman who had led many to a deepened awaraeness of their faith. Vic expressed thanks to Jill and to me for our special brand of nursing care. One of Susan's friends shared a memory of Susan that left us all with a glad heart. He described the first time he met Susan. He said that not only was she always smiling and sometimes singing, but also that she surrounded her home with flowers; "She even had flowers growing in the cracks of the driveway!"

Now, when I spend time in my garden, I look at my flowers and celebrate Susan. I celebrate her smile in the petals of the flowers; hear her laughter, kind voice, and singing in the wind; and feel her love in the sunshine. Susan cultivated a garden within me and helped me to renew my passion for nursing and healing. Thank you, Susan.

SHARING THE LAST EXPERIENCE
by Debra Butcher (Oklahoma, USA)

Nursing for me was a second career, not exactly late in life, but certainly at an age beyond that of my colleagues. I graduated the first time, at the regular college age with a degree in microbiology, having forfeited my desire to go to medical school because of marriage and following my husband's dreams. I can recall, however, my first steps into the huge auditorium at the college of nursing and knowing that I had made it at last.

During the years I took on the role of a nursing student, full-time mom, and volunteer worker, a dear friend of mine was the volunteer coordinator for a newly established hospice in our community. She would at every opportunity tell me I was destined to be a hospice nurse. I, on the other hand, declared my love for obstetrics, and that I was most certainly being led down the joy-filled path to caring for patients during labor and delivery.

After finishing school and becoming a full-fledged RN, the road to labor and delivery took quite an unexpected turn with an experience with a lovely, elderly woman named Emily.

It wasn't too far into my first year as charge nurse for the 11-7 shift that I figured out that most of our nurses did not want to sit with those who were dying. Even though I would carefully make the night assignments, somehow I would always end up parked outside a patient's room where I would wait and watch for the end to arrive. I quickly learned the value of simply being present and that nursing entailed much more than administering medications.

Emily was one of our community's unique patients whose primary physician was one of our local surgeons. Emily had known this physician when she was a young girl. Fortunately for her this was an excellent relationship, especially at this time in her life. Emily had been diagnosed with metastatic cancer, and no treatment was available considering her advanced age and fragility. This sweet and gentle lady had long outlived any relatives and now was admitted to our unit to die.

On the fourth night of my assignment, after attending to Emily's needs for relief of pain, I came onto the unit only to find her in a state of unconsciousness. The physician had left orders to adjust her pain medication as necessary to keep her comfortable. I felt sad that I could not communicate with her, but I tended to what I perceived she might need. I kept her comfortable and spoke in quiet tones to let her know I cared about what was happening to her. I kept watch over her and checked on her as often as my other patients would allow.

Several hours into the shift, as I moved past her open door, I noticed she was sitting up in bed carrying on quite a conversation with someone. Although it was late, I thought a friend had come to visit. When I entered the room, however, I saw no one there. At that time Emily let out a laugh. It was clear whoever she was conversing with was telling quite a good story.

I continued to watch this scene throughout the night as I cared for Emily and the other patients. She would often turn toward her right as if to get a better look at something or someone. She talked and laughed as though she was at a party, asking her unseen visitor to move the chair closer and reaching out her hand as if to connect with another hand. As the night turned into dawn, Emily eventually fell asleep. I softly spoke to her as I finished up my work in her room, straightening the linens, combing her hair, caring for her as if she were a close relative. I was in awe of what I thought to be a very spiritual experience and felt privileged to be a witness to her extraordinary gathering. I knew enough about nearing death that I believed when I would return for my shift later that night, her bed would be empty.

At 10:30 that evening, I walked on the unit a little sad. I just knew Emily would not be there. Instead, as I passed her room, there she sat on the edge of her bed, awake, alert, with a huge smile on her precious face. I stopped to speak to her before I made my way to the nurses' station to check in for my assignment. As I sat next to her, holding her sweet, frail hand, I asked her about the night before, about the visitors who appeared to be there but were invisible to my sight. "Why honey," she excitedly replied, "didn't you see my husband and my best friend had stopped by for a party? It was the grandest thing, talking about all of the old times. They wanted me to go home with them, but I told them I just couldn't."

Early that night, I positioned my bedside table in the hallway next to her door just as I had done the night before. Emily continued to sit on the edge of her bed occasionally letting her head fall to rest on the pillows. I checked on her about every 10 minutes, and she would arouse, smile, and tell me thanks for all I had done. Early the next morning on one of my 10-minute checks, I noticed Emily had once again leaned her shoulder and head against the pillow, resting quietly, but this time I could not see her small chest rising and falling. Coming closer to her, I could see her small hands folded as if in prayer. She had quietly left this world.

Little did I realize Emily would be one of two people who would be the guiding force that led me into hospice care. It has been many years since that night when I was honored to share in Emily's last party on this earth. For the last 7 years, I have worked in hospice, both as case manager and in administrative capacities. I have spent many days and evenings sharing and witnessing some wonderful parting moments. To be able to be present, to watch and wait, for that moment as a soul makes the journey from this world into the next is a true blessing. To know you have made a difference for someone is an affirmation to my response to the call of hospice. I truly thank Emily for the gift of her "last party" and for the difference she made in my life and in my career.

PRAYING WITH THE PATIENT
by Lindsey D. Fischer (Virginia, USA)

Childbirth is such a miraculous, spiritual event that I wanted to be a part of it. However, I had no idea I could benefit a patient so much during the labor process as I did this one patient.

I chose to work with a 21-year-old woman who was in labor with her first child. I entered the patient's room with the nurse and introduced myself as a nursing student who was there to help. She smiled in return and introduced herself as Mandy. She was an attractive young woman with blond hair and bright blue eyes. As we were conversing with each other, she would cordially smile and answer my questions with brief responses. Everything seemed fine on the surface, but behind those blue eyes I could sense anxiety and fear. She had no support person with her. When we asked Mandy if anybody would be coming, she quietly shook her head and said the father of the baby was out of town on business and that she had no family nearby. I assured her I would be there to help her in any way I could. She looked up and thanked me as I walked out of the room.

As I left the room, I thought about how difficult her situation was. She was an unmarried, soon-to-be single mom with no support person for the overwhelming laboring process. I deeply sympathized and had a strong desire to know more about her. Although she did not seem to open up to me earlier, I felt the need to return to her room. Perhaps, I thought, by taking the time to talk with Mandy I could gain her confidence and trust so she would not be afraid to talk. I thought by having her express her feelings, she might be able to relieve some of her anxiety.

I returned to the Mandy's room to try to get to know her better. She told me about her family and where she grew up. I told her about my family and my experiences in college. Mandy was a college student with a focus on elementary education. She professed her love for children but never imagined she would be in the situation she was in now: pregnant and single. I remember Mandy telling me what I must be thinking, since she was a young, unmarried soon-to-be mother. I told her I would never judge someone like that.

Mandy then told me the story of how she fell in love with the father of the baby. She met him her sophomore year of college, describing it as love at first sight. They were inseparable from that point on. The couple began to have intimate relations, and she soon found out she was pregnant. Although she was very frightened at first, she was confident her boyfriend would support her. However, when she told him about the pregnancy, he wanted her to have an abortion. In her mind, abortion was not an option, so she decided to raise the baby on her own. Her boyfriend broke up with her shortly after, and she endured the hardships of pregnancy by herself.

Mandy asked me if I thought she was doing the right thing, keeping the baby and deciding to raise it as a single parent rather than putting it up for adoption. I thought about how to answer that question. I told her only she could answer that question. Tears welled up in her eyes as she wondered how she could have gotten herself into this situation and strayed so far from the strong religious beliefs she had acquired while growing up. Mandy doubted God could still love her after the things she had done.

I will never forget telling her, "It does not matter if you do not believe in God or have lost faith or hope; God still loves you because He believes in you and will love you until the end." Tears streamed down her face. It seemed as if she had been waiting for a long time for someone to tell her that.

I asked her if she wanted me to say a prayer with her. She said, "Yes," and I began to pray that she would be comforted. I also prayed she would find the strength to make it through the labor and be able to deliver a healthy baby. Afterward, I had such a feeling of peace, knowing she was able to confide in me and find someone to console her during this experience.

Mandy's labor began to progress, and it was soon time for delivery. Although the epidural anesthesia helped with the pain, she spent a significant amount of time pushing the baby out. As Mandy prepared for her last big push, she took a big breath in and pushed as hard as she could, delivering a healthy baby girl. The beautiful baby was placed on her stomach, and she was able to embrace the infant for the first time. She immediately fell in love with the baby girl.

During the recovery period, she took my hand and thanked me for everything I had done. She said she would never forget the way I helped her and that I was exactly what she needed. That night after my clinical experience, I got on my knees and thanked God for the experience I had and the impact I was able to make on this woman. I asked the Lord to bless this new mother and the baby so she would be able to raise the child well and know she was loved.

I learned from this experience the impact nurses can have with people during life-changing experiences, from the patient fighting for life to a new baby being born. Despite the occasional frustrations nurses encounter, experiences like this make nursing unique and wonderful. Often during life-altering experiences, patients and their loved ones need a shoulder to cry on or someone to comfort them. It is important for them to know support is there.

TESTING ETHICAL PRINCIPLES IN JALIUT
by Victoria P. Niederhauser (Hawaii, USA)

We found Robbie under a mosquito net in a grass hut on the atoll of Jaliut in the Marshall Islands. He was 16 months old and weighed 10 pounds. He was weak and listless, unable to support the weight of his head. His fontanels were sunken, his lips parched, and his shiny skin had poor turgor. He had open wounds on his extremities that oozed a purulent fluid. He was unable to speak.

We were a 14-member volunteer healthcare team sent to help set up temporary clinics on remote Pacific atolls about 2,500 miles southwest of Hawaii. These atolls are very primitive, with no electricity, running water, or healthcare facilities.

Six months before we found Robbie, his parents, who lived on another atoll, decided they could no longer afford to care for him. They sent him to live with his grandparents on Jaliut. Robbie had been treated many times for failure-to-thrive at the hospital in Majuro, the largest Marshall Island.

According to the team physician who had worked in Third World countries for many years, children such as Robbie typically become ill and weaken. They no longer are able to inform others of their needs for extra fluids and food. They become lethargic and sleepy. Family members attempt to feed them until they realize food and fluid only cause more diarrhea. Thinking rest will help strengthen them, the families allow the children to sleep. Soon they realize something is terribly wrong, and they prepare to lose the child.

We quickly brought Robbie back to the clinic. The physical exam revealed 15% dehydration, severe malnutrition, and bilateral ear infection. We began oral antibiotics and oral rehydration fluids. As fast as we could get fluids into Robbie, he excreted them into his diaper. By the following morning, Robbie became more responsive and was able to hold his own bottle. We knew we had to take him from his village to the hospital. Robbie's family was reluctant to let us take him. They understood he was very sick, but they didn't trust others to care for him. After a long discussion with his family, we insisted there was no other alternative. He had to go with us to the hospital. The third day after finding him, I carried Robbie in my arms on the plane back to the hospital.

When I arrived at the hospital, the admitting pediatrician immediately recognized Robbie because of his prior admissions. He was concerned because there were no family members with him. Robbie's family could not afford the plane ride to Majuro and had no money for food and expenses if they stayed near the hospital. The hospital was very poorly staffed, and children without caretakers were often neglected. I remember the pediatrician's words clearly: "Children like this often die mysteriously in the night." I had no choice but to leave Robbie there. I placed him in a crib and headed toward the door to catch my plane back to Hawaii. As I took one final glance, Robbie extended his arms to me, as if to say, "Please don't leave me." I could not help feeling sad for Robbie, when I should have been feeling glad we had saved his life.

At the time, I did not question how we handled Robbie's situation. It wasn't until I arrived home and examined my feelings more closely that I felt confused. As nurses, we are often faced with situations that may puzzle or confuse us. We may not question an action or decision at the moment it is made, but in retrospect we may ask ourselves, "Did I do the right thing?" I couldn't help but ask myself this question over and over considering Robbie's situation.

While reviewing the process of ethical decision-making, the principle of beneficence, or the active promotion of good, was what I questioned most. Was it "good" to have saved Robbie's life knowing I might only have prolonged his suffering? The statistics indicate children with severe malnutrition have significantly lower IQ scores and a higher incidence of attention deficit. I knew Robbie would not have the opportunity to receive early intervention or special education in the Marshall Islands. Was it "good" to have taken him away from a family who loved him and place him at the mercy of strangers? Robbie had obviously suffered a great deal in his short life. Was it "good" to have interrupted an ancient lifestyle and value system in which the fittest survive? In the Marshall Islands, men are dominant figures who are viewed as strong and capable family providers. Robbie would have a lot of catching up to do to fulfill this role.

After a great deal of thought and reflection, I am able to say that if the situation arose again, I would act the same. Robbie's case provided us with the opportunity to teach the people in his village some important things. We were able to show them alternative ways to heal the sick, such as western medical actions. The dramatic changes in Robbie's responsiveness clearly demonstrated the importance of oral rehydration. Nutritional education with common island foods was also accomplished by asking the community members to prepare a rice, coconut syrup, and egg mixture for Robbie. We explained the importance of protein and potassium for children with diarrhea and dehydration.

Most importantly, Robbie's community saw a different healthcare system in action—one in which the "not so fit" can also survive. Perhaps we helped them understand something of what was possible.

The following year I returned to the Marshall Islands on a different project. I tried to find out what happened to Robbie. The hospital staff told me he was living with his parents in a remote village on Majuro. I visited the village three times and never saw Robbie. According to the village people, Robbie was with his mother at another village—she was giving birth to her second child. I visited this village, but I could not find Robbie or his family. I still wonder about him.

SUPPORTING THE PATIENT'S DETERMINATION
by Stacy L. Clark (Utah, USA)

After spending a whole year in nursing school dealing with sick patients, the idea of working with healthy women in labor during childbirth seemed more exciting. We learned all about the labor process and how naturally the baby moves into position in the uterus and descends down the birthing canal until it is expulsed from the uterus. Most babies follow the same sequence of events. Millions of deliveries take place every year. We also learned about complications that might result in a cesarean section, perhaps even death, but those events were rare. For the most part, everything happened like clockwork, and there was nothing to fear.

My first patient was an ideal patient. She was a 23-year-old, first-time mother who had a wonderful, supportive husband. She came into the labor and delivery room with contractions every few minutes. Her pregnancy had been ideal. The baby was healthy; she was also healthy. She had every reason to believe her delivery would go smoothly. She progressed at a normal pace with her cervix dilating about a centimeter every hour. Finally she heard the magical words, "You're complete!" Her cervix was completely dilated, and it was time to start pushing.

As a young student nurse, I was given the responsibility of holding one of the patient's legs and coaching her to push during each contraction. We had a great system going. As soon as the contraction monitor began to increase, her husband and I each grabbed a leg and pulled back, and the patient began to push while we all counted for 10 seconds. She would push three times, faithfully, with each contraction. She was so motivated she sometimes would throw in an extra push during a contraction, or hold pushes for an extra second. Her mom and sister were in the room too, and everyone got excited by cheering the patient on. Everyone in the room would start counting when it was time to push and would yell extra cheers and words of encouragement. After an hour and a half of pushing, we were all sure progress had been made and the baby was close to coming. After all, the textbooks explained it was normal for a first time mother to push for about 2 hours.

It was about this time that the doctor came in to check on the patient. We all waited with anticipation as he performed a pelvic exam to determine the baby's station and the progress made. Upon completion of the exam, the doctor looked up and said, "I'm afraid your baby hasn't moved a bit." An overwhelming sense of disappointment filled the room. After all that work, there was no change, and we had done everything right. We had held the legs just like we were supposed to. We used the best pushing methods, and the patient had used as much power as she could to push—yet there was no change. The doctor continued by saying, "Your baby is experiencing what we call 'failure to progress,' meaning something may be impeding his ability to descend. Keep pushing and I'll come back in 30 minutes. If the baby is still in the same position, then we'll have to go to the operating room and I'll have to remove the baby by cesarean-section."

The disappointment on everyone's faces was almost painful. From the moment this patient had walked into the room, she had stated how badly she wanted to deliver vaginally and was scared to death of having a C-section. Given the normalcy of this pregnancy, we assured her the chances of a C-section were very rare. And now, after 20 hours of labor and 1 hour of pushing, she would have to have a C-section. The doctor left, and everyone in the room was silent. Everyone appeared to be in a state of shock. However, as I looked more closely, I noticed that each head had bowed in prayer. I too bowed my head and offered a silent prayer that this young girl's efforts would not be in vain. I prayed she would be able to deliver this baby on her own without any complications. I am sure the same prayer was coming from the other four people in the room. After about 15 seconds, the silence was broken by the voice of the patient. "Come on you guys, let's get to work. We can do this!" A new type of energy filled the room as everybody assumed their respective positions. Even though this sweet girl had already exhausted herself with 90 minutes of pushing, she began to push with a type of exuberance I had never seen, not even in the best athletes. She would push four or five times per contraction and hold the pushes for at least 12 seconds. The family members were cheering louder and with more energy than before. Everyone was determined to get this baby out.

All too quickly, the 30 minutes were up. The doctor returned and we all awaited the verdict, praying more fervently than before. "The head's right here," the doctor said. "Your baby's coming!" The joy filling the room was so overwhelming we couldn't even speak. Instead, we were all moved to tears with gratitude for the miraculous outcome. Within 10 minutes, a beautiful, healthy baby boy was delivered.

Being There When Needed
by Charles Kemp (Texas, USA)

Awhile ago a former student challenged me to focus more on the eternal. I was not sure how to do this, but my respect for her is such that

I've kept it in mind waiting, I suppose, for a sign. I know that we do the work of the Samaritan, and I know there is Scriptural basis (in all religions) for such work. About a month ago we were asked to help care for Mr. S., a man with a terminal illness. Mr. S. was a Parkland patient with no insurance or Medicare. The deal we worked out was that the Parkland nurse practitioner would see him several days a week and we would go on Tuesdays and Thursdays so the Parkland NP would have a break.

Mr. S. lived with his son and daughter-in-law, their three children, his wife, and toward the end, his two sisters—all in a two-bedroom apartment in South Dallas. The daughter-in-law did nearly all the care for Mr. S., and the sisters took care of the children, cooking, and so on. What a magnificent job the daughter-in-law did! What a wonderful family.

Last Thursday we were there, changing Mr. S.'s dressings and getting him cleaned up. By this point he had gangrene in both feet and pneumonia, and the cardiac insufficiency that brought him to this point was worsening. Clearly he was close to death. As always, when we finished with the physical care, we had a prayer with Mr. S. and his family. Lupe (the Agape promotora) prayed with us and for us, and as always, we were touched. Mr. S. died at home that night. I thought about the time we spent with Mr. S., and especially the last day and the last prayer. That was an eternal thing!

OVERCOMING BARRIERS
by Terri Harder (Florida, USA)

I met Mrs. K in November 1998. She was 19 years old and a newlywed, had two daughters ages 3 and 4, was pregnant, and had recently been diagnosed with HIV. She was new to the Naples area and spoke two languages—English wasn't one of them. With the assistance of a translator, I introduced her to the Healthy Start program (a state-funded program that assists pregnant women in obtaining necessary resources to improve the health of newborn babies and to reduce the infant mortality rate).

At our first meeting, I discussed client confidentiality and explained the translator was also bound to uphold the code of confidentiality. I explained the importance of attending all appointments at the obstetrical and infectious disease clinics and encouraged her to take all her prescribed medicines. After completing my initial assessment, I knew this would be a challenging family to manage.

I discovered several barriers to obtaining healthcare for Mrs. K., such as the lack of a home telephone, a lack of transportation, and the language barrier. I also discovered she wasn't eligible for Medicaid and had no funds to pay for her healthcare or prescriptions. I worked with the staff in the infectious disease office helping Mrs. K apply for emergency medical funds, which resulted in deferring the charges associated with some of the medical appointments and the transportation fees to attend these appointments. Referrals were made to WIC (a supplemental food and nutrition program for pregnant women and children). I also reviewed the immunization records for the girls and escorted them to the immunization clinic after Mrs. K attended a clinic appointment.

I wanted to schedule well-child exams with a pediatrician for the children, but without Medicaid, that was difficult. In an attempt to assist Mrs. K in applying for Medicaid for the girls, I discovered they didn't have birth certificates or social security numbers. After several telephone calls to the Office of Vital Statistics, the Social Security Administration, and the Clerk of Civil courts, this issue was resolved.

As time went by, Mrs. K wasn't attending all her scheduled appointments. She should have run out of her antiretroviral medication, so I assumed she wasn't taking the medicine as prescribed. This resulted in several attempts at follow-up home visits. Mrs. K denied having adverse side effects from the medicine, so again, I reinforced the importance of taking the medicine in the hopes that her baby would be born healthy. Mrs. K continued to miss scheduled appointments and hadn't refilled her prescription, so I asked nurses from the infectious disease clinic to accompany me on a home visit. Another staff member came along as a Spanish translator. Previously I used a Creole translator. I thought I was being sensitive to my client's cultural differences by asking members of the same cultural community as my patient to act as my translators, but I learned the Spanish translator was welcomed more readily.

I thought I had resolved all the problems and that things would run smoothly from here on out. Mrs. K now had a home telephone so it would be easier to contact her. Unfortunately, she continued to miss appointments, so I continued to make home visits. Finally we did meet up after a period of time. I told Mrs. K that there were other people who could use my help, so I was going to close her case. I said I wouldn't be telephoning her or stopping by the house anymore, but I gave her my business card and asked her to call me if she needed anything. She began to cry. She said she wanted my help. As the tears flowed, so did her thoughts. Will my baby be okay? She was talking to me in broken English!

Mrs. K was in a "catch 22." Her husband was a spiritual man and told her "God came to me in a dream and you are no longer sick." She rationalized she didn't need her medicine any more. She wanted to please her husband but was worried her baby would be born with "the virus." We discussed the difference between HIV and AIDS and the fact that she may live a long time if she took care of herself. I told her I couldn't argue with God, but stated since the doctor had previously found the virus in her blood, she should take the medicine. She agreed to take it.

Five weeks later, Mrs. K had a baby boy. I reinforced the importance of his being monitored by the doctors in our clinic for 18-24 months. I accompanied the family to the pediatrician appointment to provide Mrs. K's prenatal history because she had a habit of saying "yes" to most questions.

I worked closely with her the next 2 months and explained a new nurse was going to be the baby's nurse and would coordinate all of his appointments to the pediatrician and immunology. I gave her my card and told her to call me anytime if she needed me. Over the next few weeks, I made several attempts to give her a bag of clothes for her little girls, but I never found anyone at home. Her new nurse did visit her and finally gave her the clothes. The following week I received a telephone call from Mrs. K thanking me for the clothes.

Currently, Mrs. K is at home with the children during the day and is employed during the evenings. The baby is now chubby, happy, and thriving. He'll continue to see the pediatric immunologist. I think of this family often. Although the case has been closed, I find myself driving by the house hoping to see Mrs. K or one of the children, and when I do see them, I am always greeted with hugs and kisses.

CULTURAL CONFIDENCES
by Laura A. Barry (Massachusetts, USA)

As a new grad, I knew I had a lot to learn. Some of my knowledge came from one of my patients, a young man who was dying. I will always be grateful to him because he taught me so much medically, culturally, and emotionally.

This patient was a young Chinese man who was dying of a brain lymphoma. AIDS further complicated his medical status. As you can surmise, his medical treatment was quite involved. That in itself provided a welcomed learning experience, but what he taught me about culture, family love, and pride was enlightening.

His medical regimen was complicated. It consisted of many medications that were unfamiliar to me. An IV bolus here, premedications there. His medications were so complicated that I wondered if I would ever get the hang of being a nurse?

The patient's family was very supportive. His mother rubbed his limbs with ancient Chinese preparations. There was at least one family member in his room at almost all times. One night he took the opportunity, while we were alone, to tell me that his family was unaware of his terminal status. He explained that in the Chinese culture, this would be considered a weakness. He asked me not to tell anyone in his family of his diagnosis. My heart ached to let them know so that they could support him. However, other team members and I were bound to silence because of patient confidentiality. My knowledge of his culture was limited, which led to great frustration on my part. There were tears in my eyes as I explained my concerns to him. He patted my hand and told me to be strong. In spite of the circumstances, he was comforting me!

His candidness with me led to many open conversations, and I felt I was fulfilling the "big sister" role. I was grateful. He felt he could talk to me and didn't always have to be the stoic one. I, thankfully, had many resources and people to talk to. There were clinical educators, senior staff, and ancillary staff to help me. I was grateful to them for helping me carry the load. My nurse manager even complimented me for "taking on such a challenging patient."

As the patient's health deteriorated, he began to refuse his medications. This brought on a whole new set of issues. My job was not to judge but to support. This was the most difficult aspect of nursing I had encountered. Why couldn't he see that he needed to take his medications? My heart broke as he explained that he had come to terms with his terminal status and was ready. His wish was to go home to die. Countless meetings with pastoral care, social services, and hospice care ensued. None, however, of the participants included his family members. He held fast to his desire to keep his illnesses from his family.

He was discharged to home and I never heard from him again. We read of his death in the paper a few weeks later. I will never know if he ever let his family in on his secrets or what his final days were like. I only hope I was able to somehow make as much of a difference in his life as he made in mine.

In the early morning hours, while the world is asleep, nurses care for and watch over patients. It is frequently a still and almost sacred time. There is prayer and reflection. Rooms have bits and pieces of religious symbols and icons. In honor of their religions, families share their rituals and reflect with quiet meditations and prayer incantations. All the while, nurses watch and participate—as they can and as they are asked to. Nurses support families in many ways. Among those ways is the honoring of diverse religious practices; the participation in religious practices as time and situations allow; and the everyday belief that their work is part of a larger plan.

REFERENCES

Black, J., Hawks, J., & Keene, A. (2001). Medical-surgical nursing. Clinical management for positive outcomes (6th ed.). Philadelphia: W.B. Saunders.

Brigham Young University College of Nursing. (2002). *The Healer's Art.* Provo, UT.

Boutell, K.A., & Bozett, E.W. (1987). Nurses assessment of patient spirituality: Continuing education implications. Journal of Continuing Education, 21(4), 172-176.

Lemmer, C. (2002). Teaching the spiritual dimension of nursing care: A Survey of U.S. baccalaureate nursing programs. Journal of Nursing Education, 41(11), 482-491.

Swearingen, P., & Ross, D. (1999). Manual of medical-surgical nursing care (4th ed.). St. Louis, MO: Moby, Inc.

Spector, R.E. (2004). Cultural diversity in health and illness (6th ed.). Newark, NJ: Pearson Prentice Hall.

Weaver, A.J., Flannelly, L.T., & Flannelly, K.J. (2001). A review of research on religious and spiritual variable in two primary gerontological nursing journals: 1991 to 1997. Journal of Gerontological Nursing, 27(9), 48-54.

I am grateful to A. Elaine Bond and the stories submitted for *The Healers' Art,* Anniversary Celebration. Written by students and colleagues at Brigham Young University, many of these beautiful stories grace this chapter. I am privileged to acknowledge and share their work with you.

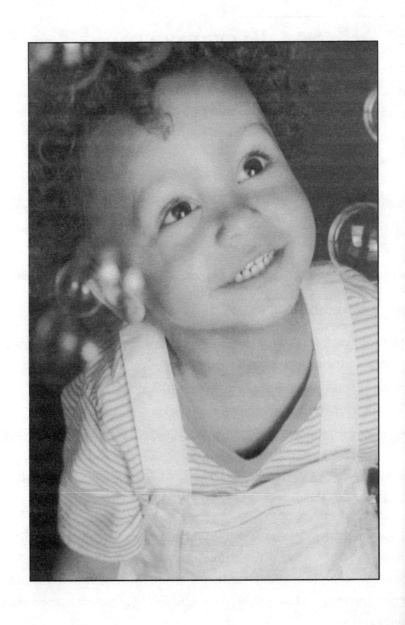

CHAPTER 5

Being There: Caring in the Community

Mindprint

I live in a world that no one knows,
a world known only to me.
It holds my soul,
my realm of storied truths
that shape my destiny.

—*by June Heider Bisson*

Nursing in the community is a tangled web of healthcare net-works. It is a well-traveled alley behind rickety houses with broken front porches. It is a foot-worn path to a trailer home, lined with plas-tic flowers and six barking dogs. It's a beat public health nurses trav-el from home to home with trunks full of supplies—a system that is difficult to navigate, unless you care to know how.

This type of nursing is perhaps the oldest form of nursing, dating back to the 1870s. Pioneers Lillian Wald and Mary Brewster opened New York City's Henry Street Settlement House in the late 1890s for those who needed care, whether they could pay or not. This type of nursing led the field in World War I and the Great Depression of the 1930s (Drevdahl, Kneipp, Canales, & Dorcy, 2001; Leddy & Pepper, 1998). The practices and beliefs of these historic nurse heroes con-tinue to thrive in public health nursing today.

Community nursing is sometimes called public health nursing. The settings are as diverse as the people the nurses serve. Community health nursing occurs in the home, with the nurse traveling from point to point. The goal is to care for patients in their own settings, their comfort zones, their homes.

The home may be a high-rise, apartment, low-income center, or suburban dwelling. The home may be a homeless shelter or a hospice dwelling. The home may be someone's car or a spot under a bridge. It may be in the deepest inner city or on a remote island. It takes great maturity, experience, and decision-making abilities to be a nurse in the community. These nurses are often the only healthcare providers for the patients. They make swift, life-saving decisions. Often their patients are found quite ill, unresponsive, in desperate need of care. Ask a community health nurse how many times she or he has done CPR in the home, and the answer will be "too many times." Ask a public health nurse how many times she or he has called 911, the numbers are staggering. Every day there is a lonely elderly person who needs home care. It is the nurse who assesses, plans, and treats patients daily in the home, whatever home might be for that person. It is the nurse who travels in every type of weather (sometimes in a plane or small motorboat) to assist children who are hemophiliacs and live in isolated locations. Nurses are concerned about their patients, knowing full well that many patients can't make it without care for even one night. Realizing that a patient may be ventilator-dependent and in need of pulmonary hygiene, the nurse's SUV goes full-speed ahead.

Community nursing is different from hospital-based nursing. The demand for skills and the challenges are certainly there, but these trailblazers are up to the task. Finding a patient with a dangerously low heart rate as a result of beta blocker drugs (prescribed but not closely monitored) and correcting the problem is rewarding. Forestalling diabetic coma in a diabetic patient with perilously low blood sugars is life saving. The rewards are frequent, but so are the risks.

As the nurse gingerly enters the home setting, there is no telling what will be found. Nurses overcome scores of obstacles and time and again risk their own lives (unknowingly) when they provide home care. Domestic squabbles are all too common, as is violence. Guns, pimps, and prostitution are part of the scene. Nurses need courage administering care to patients living in rooms that are studded with bullet holes. They need courage when the smell of gun smoke wafts in the air while a sweet baby smiles in a nearby crib. They need courage when a boa constrictor snake is the family pet.

Sometimes the patients don't want to be helped. Telling people what they "ought to do" is unpopular for sure. Telling people what they "must do" may get you thrown out of the house. These are people who are down on their luck, unemployed, and impacted by a myriad of negative forces, many of them beyond their control as individuals. Many nurses realize they need to be advocates for the poor and recognize the limits and barriers in the community. They are proponents for healthcare for all and live this motto every day. Unfortunately they need to deal with social boundaries and a health-care system that is often unjust and disorganized. Equally depressing is the presence of racism and biased and uninformed attitudes.

Advocacy, activism, and investigation are the words that describe community healthcare. Why is it that all the painkillers are gone after only 4 postoperative days? Why is it that the lead levels are so high in these children as compared to the standards, the norms? Are those cigarette burns on the toddler's face and mouth? Every single family member has pulmonary TB that is resistant to antibiotics. How did it get so bad? The mother said she was raped by a boyfriend. Excrement is everywhere and so are beer bottles, drug paraphernalia, and strangers. And the most startling fact, the most disturbing point of reference, is that the children are playing through it all. The children are unfazed because it is their world, their bad world. How did all of this happen and who cares about these people?

The nurse in the community is the detective and the primary care-taker. It is these nurses who care about the children, the mothers, the elderly. It is these nurses who give rides in their own cars to a 70-year-old man who cannot get from Dr. A to Dr. B. It is these nurses who bring a meal, give childhood immunizations, and screen refugees every day. First hand, they treat acute problems such as ear infections, pharyngitis, and skin problems. They monitor chronic conditions—diabetes, hypertension, asthma, and obesity. They integrate nursing and cultural competency, make follow-up visits, teach health-related classes, and identify the risks in their communities. Most of all, they make sure no one falls through the healthcare cracks.

Their work is humble yet vital, expeditious yet caring, limit-setting yet heartfelt. From the elderly in the high-rise who look forward to the company and medical attention to the child with a severe untreated fungal infection, it is the nurse who is at the bedside in the home preventing disaster and restoring health. They boldly go where no one has gone before. They boldly go where no one wants to go.

TAKING STEPS IN ANOTHER'S SHOES
by Nancy Hartley (Florida, USA)

Thirteen years ago I had an African-American patient named Greg. He was a drug addict living with his mother and two other siblings. The family had no car so transportation was a problem. The mother had a minimum-wage job at a state facility.

Greg said he wanted to get off drugs, so the social worker and I called local drug rehab centers trying to get him admitted. His lack of insurance and the long waiting lists at each drug treatment center resulted in his being discharged back home. I suggested he attend Narcotics Anonymous (NA) meetings as an alternative to the rehab. Again transportation was a problem, so I volunteered to drive him to his first meeting if he would attend NA meetings. He attended a meeting but unfortunately was not truly committed to giving up his drug habit and always had a reason for not attending another meeting. To learn to overcome an addiction, one must really want to overcome it or any attempts are useless. I experienced firsthand the manipulation, broken promises, strained relationships, and multitude of other human dynamics that go with being a family member, friend, or counselor of a drug addict. I still find it difficult to balance being compassionate and yet not being a "patsy" with those who have addictions. My psychiatric experience in nursing school did not even begin to prepare me for the skills needed when working with a drug addict. Time and again there were disappointments, and I considered giving up, but I could not give up the belief that sometime, somewhere, and in some way I might reach him and convince him to give up drugs.

His mother, long frustrated by his drug addiction and her inability to stop it, often called me for help and advice. As a result Ms. C, as her co-workers called her, and I became good friends. Through that friendship I became aware of what it is like to have no transportation and the daily struggles that result from not having a car. Watching her trying to get to work at night, finding a ride to the grocery store, or keeping a doctor's appointment made me realize the obstacles my patients faced outside the hospital. I learned that we healthcare providers do not always have realistic expectations for discharge planning because we are unaware of the obstacles the patients must deal with. Further, many are proud and do not want their difficulties known. I now try to be sensitive to the barriers that would keep patients from carrying out discharge plans.

As I visited the housing project, I saw many teenagers with nothing to do and the resulting tendency to get into trouble. I saw the sale and use of drugs. This was not anything like the middle class environment where I grew up. Now as patients come into the emergency room from these housing projects, I have a better understanding of the culture in which they live. Having money to do laundry was sometimes a struggle for my friend and her family, and on occasion I would take laundry to my house and do it for them. This impressed another young Black woman a great deal and she said to me, "I never saw a White person doing laundry for Black people before."

Such actions often provided a bridge for new relationships with those who saw White people as their enemies or people not to be trusted. In my subsequent years of working as an emergency room nurse, I have often been able to diffuse angry situations because of that understanding.

Ms. C is often asked for help by her neighbors and friends. She is known for her generosity and understanding nature. This has often resulted in her asking me to help in situations where my nursing expertise is needed. One such time was when a toddler in the housing project was placed in a tub of extremely hot water and his feet and groin area were burned and blistered. The mother of the toddler did not want to take him to the hospital. After seeing the severity of the burns, I was able to convince her he needed medical attention so we took him to the hospital for treatment.

Surviving the demands of the welfare system causes many to have fear and distrust of those in authority. This often makes it difficult for them to seek medical care when needed. Sometimes it results in them being less than truthful when speaking with healthcare providers. I now try to do small things that show concern and respect to earn their trust.

Greg was frequently arrested as a result of his drug habit. I occasionally visited Greg with his family at the jail. There were times when Greg and his family felt the correctional officers at the jail were not professional in their responses to inmates. Thus when an opening was announced for membership on the County Advisory Board for the Department of Corrections, I applied and was accepted.

In the approximate 5 years that I served on the board, including a term as chairperson, I saw a new jail built and healthcare contracted out to a private firm. Twice I was asked to serve on the committee to review and rate the submitted proposals from firms seeking the health-care contract. I became much more aware of the issues inmates often experienced regarding their healthcare. The knowledge I gained from this volunteer work was often helpful as a nurse in the emergency room when we planned for the discharge of an inmate back to the jail. I was aware of the difficulties and limitations of healthcare at the jail.

When the new jail was built, and prior to inmate habitation, I even participated in a sleepover at the jail with selected community members. I was very grateful for the "get out of jail free" pass that I possessed during the sleepover. I still get a headache when I remember the hard pillow I was given to sleep on that night.

Ms. C struggled to keep her other son and daughter in school and out of trouble—a task not made easy while living in the housing project. Thus one year, as she contemplated what to do with her income tax refund check, I encouraged her to check into buying a home in the city program that allowed low-income families to purchase homes. She was able to qualify for the program and soon found herself moving into a duplex home as an owner.

This proved to be a turning point for her younger son and daughter as they were removed from the influence of crime, drugs, and promiscuity at the housing project. Unfortunately, neither of them finished high school, but both are now employed and productive citizens. Both Ms. C and I hope that someday they will pursue their GEDs and perhaps even consider a college education. But we're grateful they were removed from that environment in time to avoid being drawn into the life of crime and drugs.

Ms. C has several chronic health problems, even though she is employed and has insurance. As a minimum wage earner, simply paying the deductible for healthcare or the cost of medication can be a problem and can result in a prescription not being filled or a visit to the doctor being unattainable. So often we healthcare providers think if a person has insurance with a drug plan there is no problem affording the medications. Yet co-pays can often exceed the budget of even those with a regular income. Now I try to be aware of those limitations and find alternatives or make the physicians aware of the costs even with insurance. And I don't find myself so judgmental when patients come in with problems as a result of not having taken medications because they couldn't afford them.

Little did I know, when I had Greg as a patient many years ago, that I would take a journey into cultural diversity, visit jails, experience the waiting room of the health department, experience life in the housing projects, or encounter the multitude of other experiences I've had as a result of my friendship with his family. I believe that I have made their life better in many ways, but they too have made me a better person and a better nurse. It's as though I have taken a few steps in another's shoes and have gained a great deal of understanding that I would never have had otherwise.

DOING HUMANITARIAN WORK IN MEXICO
by Sandra Mangum (Utah, USA)

Humanitarian work has to be one of the most meaningful ways to give of self and follow the example of the Savior. I have made six trips so far—three to Mexico and three to Guatemala—as part of a plastic surgery team, Hirsche Smiles Foundation. The team consists of a surgeon, an assistant, two anesthesiologists, perioperative and recovery room nurses, and students. The goal of the team is to help children and adults who cannot afford or lack access to the surgical care they need for birth deformities such as cleft lips and palates, microtia, polydactylism, and for injuries such as burns.

As we arrive at the hospital, the waiting room is filled with parents and more than 100 children, some of whom have walked or traveled by bus for hours for the opportunity to be seen. They wait their turn to be evaluated and are either chosen for surgery or sent home disappointed. Those whose deformities are too complex to be done in their country are referred to an agency for possible transport to Utah. Some children appear for a second surgery wearing their dirty and tattered Hirsche Smiles T-shirts from the year before. The children with cleft lips and palates are always first priority. We schedule ten to twelve surgeries per day and announce to the waiting parents which child is scheduled on which day.

Busy days follow as we bathe the children, set up the operating rooms, clean and sterilize instruments, perform the surgeries, give immediate postoperative care, and educate the parents regarding oral antibiotics, pain medications, etc. The nurse liaison works with the native nurses to make sure the children are well cared for during the night. Somehow, miraculously, we are able to communicate in Spanish, at least enough to have open dialogue with the native nurses, visiting surgeons, medical students, parents, and children.

As the week progresses and we count the remaining surgeries and make sure the number of needed supplies will be adequate, we always seem to have OR packs and IV solutions left over. We remember and understand the Biblical parable of the loaves and the fishes in a broader context.

We work non-stop from early morning to late at night, sleep very little, and rise again the next morning to do the same thing again. And miraculously, rather than turn some children away whom we could help given enough energy, supplies, and time, we are able to stretch our own energy to its maximum and go beyond what seems humanly possible to help the children. We are given the blessing of "strength beyond our own."

We also have the opportunity to touch the lives of the native medical team members who observe the surgeries. They are invited to join in our prayer, given in either Spanish or English, as we ask for a special blessing for each child before the surgery begins.

Most of all, our hearts fill with joy and peace each time we take a child back to the parents. Their tears flow as they see their child for the first time whole, beautiful, and safe. Our tears flow, too, as mothers cover their children with kisses and turn to say, "God bless you for coming. You are an answer to our prayers."

OPENING THE DOORS TO DISCUSSION
by Margaret "Peggy" Patton (North Carolina, USA)

In the early 1970s, about 5 years after my graduation from a baccalaureate nursing program, I was working as a public health nurse in a county outside of New York City. It was in that position that I met the patient who changed my perspective on many aspects of life and death.

Tommy was 17 years old and well-known in the community as the golden boy with a soccer ball. Every college that had a varsity soccer team was recruiting him. He was enjoying all the attention his senior year in high school when tragedy struck. He had pain in his left leg and a small area that wouldn't heal. It didn't get better; it got worse. It took only a few weeks and the doctors got him to admit that he had been having pain for several weeks before the sore. He was diagnosed with a malignant sarcoma in his left femur. After treatment efforts of chemotherapy and radiation were attempted with no evidence of success, a left hemipelvectomy was performed, and his left leg and half of his pelvis were removed.

Now the fight focused on living rather than saving his limb. But the postoperative treatment was to no avail. Tommy's prognosis was death. His family was adamant he should not know this, and they took him home. His condition deteriorated much quicker than the family had expected, and they were running out of cheerleader answers that he was getting better. The mother turned to sedatives, the father to alcohol, and the younger daughter was totally out of control—and no one was talking to Tommy. Private duty nurses were hired to respond to Tommy's care needs. They came around the clock every 8 hours; they became his link with life. He was kept in his upstairs bedroom, being turned from supine to prone and back again, with his left side held up by a pillow. He was fed, bathed, and toileted on a bedpan.

At this point in the story, a neighbor telephoned the county health department to try to seek some help for the family. Since I was the nurse for that area of the county, the call was given to me. The neighbor told me the story and begged that someone would "do something to help this family."

I telephoned the doctor the neighbor believed was the family's physician and was met with a pitiful response that there wasn't anything anyone could do, but if I wanted to visit to go ahead. I was to absolutely not tell Tommy of his impending demise. The family did not want the topic discussed.

A very inebriated, middle-aged man met me at the door of the house and told me to go upstairs, but not to mention anything about his son's prognosis or I "would answer" to him. I walked into a foul-smelling, dark room with a figure lying on a rumpled bed of dirty sheets and a large woman sitting on a chair in the corner, sleeping. I was greeted with a very surly, "What the @#$##@#$ do you want?" from the figure in the bed. I introduced myself to the boy in the bed and requested that the nurse in the corner go downstairs for a while and get a cup of coffee. I spent the first few minutes telling Tommy I was the nurse who always worked in that town and that I had heard he and his family were having some problems. He accepted this and then turned his head from his pillow to say, "I suppose you are going to tell me that I'll be okay, like everybody else. Won't anyone have the guts to tell me that I am dying?" He was very quiet. I was paralyzed. I didn't know what to say. He was begging for someone to be honest with him, and I was sworn to secrecy. I finally knelt down by the side of his bed and quietly said to him, "Tommy, if you know that you are dying, why do you need someone to tell you? Tell me what you know; I promise I will listen."

We hugged and cried and talked and listened for about 2 hours. At the end of the 2 hours, I bathed him and changed the bed. I opened windows and generally cleaned his environment. Leaving him propped up in bed with a drink, I left promising to return tomorrow. He told me that coming back tomorrow would not be necessary; that what I had done for him today was enough. He smiled at me and with a hug said, "Thank you for letting me know the truth."

I drove the 30 minutes back to the office. After I had been there for about an hour and a half, I received a telephone call, again from the caring neighbor, telling me that Tommy had died about an hour ago. He had asked for his parents to come to his room and told them that he loved them and he was okay and as they all hugged together, Tommy died peacefully in his parents' arms.

I have always remembered this young man as one of the most poignant cases I have ever had the opportunity to be a part of. It is my conviction, from Tommy and others with whom I have shared their last moments, that no one dies without knowing it. We all need to share this knowledge and experience. If a family cannot face the death of a loved one alone, it may be the job of the nurse to help the patient and the family deal with their burden. I will always remember Tommy.

Many nurses say they feel like investigators—the Sherlock Holmes of healthcare. Armed with a keen eye, just plain good intuition, and tons of common sense, they ask the hard questions and find the answers, even if the answers mean taking hard stances. It is not okay to accept elevated lead levels no matter what the insurance covers for a child. Elevated is elevated. It is not okay to watch abuse and let it continue. The abuser must be stopped.

Nurses teach and protect. They know of the many rumors out there about HIV, not to mention the social isolation of this disease. They are there to inform, educate, and translate information into terms more easily understood. They are armed with the power of intuition, activism, and concern for the lives of many. Powerful tools for powerful men and women who care for others.

BEING PERSISTENT, ASSERTIVE, AND PREVENTATIVE
by Gwendolyn F. Foss (South Carolina, USA)

When working as a staff public health nurse, I received a referral from a pediatrician who had found elevated lead levels in a Hmong infant whose family did not speak English. When I visited the family, I discovered an extended family of 18 living in a house adjacent to an old commercial landfill. This group included a pregnant girl, five children under the age of 5 years, and several sets of parents and grandparents. The family grew its own vegetables in the yard around the house. Over the next month, I worked with various state and local agencies to have the soil surrounding the house tested and blood samples obtained from all family members for lead level testing. All family members had markedly elevated blood lead levels. The soil around the house contained high levels of lead and other heavy metals. As a result of the soil analysis, the house was condemned. After many additional home visits with an interpreter, I explained the dangers of lead, the route of exposure, and respective roles and responsibilities of various community agencies regarding lead issues and the family's safety. As a result of these meetings, the family stopped eating the food grown in the yard, applied for and received alternate housing, and agreed to treatment of family members with dangerously high blood levels of lead. In essence, I was able to prevent further occurrences of lead poisoning in that family and to prevent anyone else from living in a house and environment that contained heavy metals.

USING NATURAL RESOURCES IN MALAWI
by Nancy L. Fahrenwald (South Dakota, USA)

When I think of Africa, I think of mangos. This sweet, juicy fruit grows in the dry season, a time when few other plants thrive. Mr. M, RN, was my Malawian counterpart in the effort to plan and implement AIDS prevention and control programs for the Zomba district, a mountainous area consisting of the community of Zomba and remote villages within the country of Malawi in southern Africa. Our efforts focused on identifying high-risk populations for transmission of HIV, such as prisoners, soldiers, and prostitutes. We focused on developing home-based care and hospital-based counseling and care programs for people with AIDS. Implementing primary prevention programs in schools throughout the district of 650,000 people was a top priority.

In an effort to reach the most rural villages, we developed village AIDS committees with the permission and blessing of the village chiefs. The village AIDS committees were the primary source of HIV and AIDS information and resources for the people. Committee members were trained on HIV/AIDS transmission prevention strategies, as well as on care for people with AIDS. Reaching the rural villagers was our challenge. We had no transportation. My Peace Corps-issued bicycle was very helpful within a 15-mile radius of Zomba, where I lived, but beyond 15 miles, the villages were too remote to reach in a day's bicycle ride.

On one occasion, the Malawi education coordinator for UNICEF gave us access to her Landrover. Mr. M and I piled into the back of the vehicle, and the driver traversed bumpy, narrow, mountainous roads for nearly 2 hours so that we could train a rural village's AIDS committee. It was the hot season. Dust blew and temperatures soared. I was miserable. Homesick thoughts overcame me, despite the rewarding and challenging work with which I had been blessed. When we reached the village, the committee members were hungry. We shared the Coca-Cola and biscuits we always supplied at these trainings. I knew that this food was perhaps all the people had to eat that day.

The village chief challenged us that day. He asked us to work with the village but to also realize that he, too, needed help. His six sons and their wives were all dead. He was left to care for 17 grandchildren. He was too old to farm the soil. He couldn't grow enough food or supply school fees for the children. The children hadn't eaten that day or the day before. Our educational efforts became relief efforts, as we struggled to identify basic subsistence resources that could be shared with the chief, his family, and other villagers who were in the same situation. The crisis of AIDS was very real that day, and I was overwhelmed.

On the bumpy return ride, I cried. My tears were for the villagers and for myself. Thoughts of home came to me again; I was extremely hot, thirsty, and very hungry. I felt discouraged and powerless to change the situation in the village. Suddenly, Mr. M shouted a question, "Isn't God wonderful?" I was thinking differently. He pointed to a woman sitting under the shelter of a mango tree located along the isolated rural road. He exclaimed, "God has given us the mango so that we have at least something to put in our stomachs when nothing else will grow."

The blessing of the mango is a story of faith, belief in the unimaginable, and hope for a better world. I was no longer thinking of home. I was no longer hungry, hot, or thirsty, and I never refused a mango again.

COLLABORATING TO BENEFIT PATIENTS
by Gwendolyn F. Foss (South Carolina, USA)

As part of my job as a staff public health nurse, I was able to help one of the families in my caseload reunite with the wife's mother and brother from Vietnam. They had been unable to leave until the development of the Family Unification Program, in which Vietnam allowed selected individuals to legally leave the country, making it possible for them to join their family. The 21-year-old brother had an uncorrected cleft lip and palate. For all of his life in Vietnam, he had been sequestered in his house, without access to healthcare and education. When he arrived in the U.S., he was penniless and only had refugee benefits for a short time. By working with several community agencies, medical groups, and hospitals, I was able to arrange corrective surgery with subsequent extensive speech therapy for him. After recovery and completion of his therapy, people could understand his speech. Only a small scar on his upper lip remained. This cleft palate repair made it possible for him to attend English as a Second Language (ESL) classes and begin a path toward obtaining a job and living an independent life. His status in the Vietnamese community changed from someone who was shunned to a person who was an accepted community participant.

Nursing in the home leads to unbelievable relationships. Sometimes connections occur when nurses least expect them. In a housing project, a 25-year-old mother of five is trying her best to lead a good life. The nurse is there to help. Drugs, gangs, guilt by association, condemnation, and ridicule are what this young mother faces every day.

It is not okay to judge a mother struggling to survive in a housing project as incompetent when she is trying her best. It is certainly not okay to listen to dispatchers joke and laugh about a fire that occurred in that same setting. What nurses see, hear, and remember lead to such sorrow, they cannot forget, ever. In a troubled housing project, nurses do their best. In a world that no one seems to care about, it is the nurse who adds clarity. That is greatness, taking the time to hear what is going on in troubled parts of the world. The following story beckons us to be aware of our own prejudices. The story is revolting because one of the worst aspects of social injustice is revealed: institutionalized racism.

MAKING CONNECTIONS
by Elizabeth A. Tyree (North Dakota, USA)

At the time of this story, I worked as a maternal and child health specialist for Elgin County, which surrounded a medium-large city, Napier. The city and county health departments were separate, as were most of the government and service agencies. I worked with different caseloads of high-risk children every year: those who had been in infant intensive care; families where abuse was a problem; and families that were headed by parents with mental retardation. My purpose was to develop standards of care and prepare the public health nurses to serve these populations.

At the time of this event I was assigned a neighborhood area outside the city limits, which had the characteristics of an inner city ghetto with a high crime rate, gangs, prostitution, drugs, and violence. There were several housing projects in which these problems were pervasive, and none more so than Sunrise Circle.

Sunrise Circle was notorious, including one incident where residents beat a police officer with a smoldering outdoor grill filled with charcoal. The police went in with force, six squad cars at a time. The Salvation Army and Goodwill refused to make deliveries to Sunrise Circle, as did other merchants. My entree was to work with high-risk infants, but my role expanded to serve the whole family as best I could. I was as affected as anyone might be by the daily news and scenes of mayhem at any of the housing projects, but particularly Sunrise Circle. When I visited Sunrise Circle, I parked near the gated entrance, to minimize exposing my car to random acts of vandalism, and had my purse locked in the trunk. Since my reason for being there was to help high-risk infants, I walked in carrying a baby scale; sometimes past the gang of young men; sometimes through the police line. I was not so naive as to think I would be so accepted that I would not ever be subject to violence myself. I knew it could happen, but thought people would have a hard time arguing with a baby scale.

I met Darla under these circumstances. She was at her mother's townhouse in Sunrise Circle and had recently given birth to Nathan. She was 25 and this was her fifth child. She thought she had done something right by having her tubes tied after this baby. Her other children were Ethan, 12 years old; Lawrence, 10; Denise, 3; and Unice, 2. Denise and Unice liked to prance like carousel ponies around in a circle, as preschoolers often do. Ethan was big and husky for 12 years. Baby Nathan was healthy and gaining weight. Darla and I agreed I would visit periodically and that she would take the little children to the Women, Infants, and Children (WIC) nutrition program and begin Nathan's immunizations. It was easy to engage Darla. She seemed genuinely interested in her children and doing well as a mother.

Through Darla I met her mother, Betsy. Betsy was 64. She had arthritis and hypertension. She wasn't receiving medical care. The family had only recently moved to Sunrise Circle from a very big city not far away. I visited Betsy periodically getting to know her, arranging for her to be treated for her hypertension and arthritis. I knew her fondest dream was to have a beautifully decorated, flocked Christmas tree, and all of her children and grandchildren around it. Perhaps the new start she and her family were making in Napier would lead to the realization of this dream. I also knew she had an 18-year-old son, but according to the housing authority, he couldn't live with Betsy. Even though she had two bedrooms in her townhouse, he was no longer classified as a dependent and had to be on his own.

Darla moved her family into a townhouse across the court from Betsy. Furniture was sparse, but gradually Darla made a home for them.

She bought goose-patterned kitchen accessories and Contac paper, which she used to wallpaper the kitchen walls. It didn't work so well, though, and started peeling off. She bought fancy living room furniture on a delayed payment plan from the cut-rate furniture store, which started to look the worse for wear when food was rubbed into the "fine" upholstery.

We did some good things together. I helped Darla take advantage of a Christmas toy give-away, and we hauled a carload of toys back to Gramma's for Christmas surprises. I carried Nathan through the WIC clinic while Darla managed Denise and Unice for the blood tests, heights, and weights, even though I couldn't keep up with his diarrhea, and my dress was soaked. I even drove them in my car, not to mention the fact I didn't have car seats. I even counseled Darla's pimp about his skin rash.

On March 13, I had an appointment to visit Darla at ten o'clock. That was my first appointment of the day since I would be working through the dinner hour with a mother who was mentally retarded and had a 5-year-old daughter with encopresis, retaining stool. Someone from the office called to warn me that there had been a fire at Sunrise Circle and there had been children involved, in case I hadn't heard the news. I asked for the address, and it wasn't Darla's. So I went.

Walking into Sunrise Circle was nothing like it had ever been. Fire and police workers were still there. Coming closer, I could see it was Darla's apartment that had burned. It had rained over night and there was a lot of mud around. Two of the mothers I knew came running up to me and said, "They just threw those babies in the mud. They didn't care. Ethan was calling from the top of the stairs, 'Help! Help!' and they wouldn't go up there and help him. Thirty minutes we waited for the fire trucks. They won't help us. They won't send an ambulance in here." A news reporter shoved a microphone in my face, which I pushed away. The racial makeup of the crowd said it all. The residents were all Black and the news people, firemen, police, and I were all White. I had nothing to offer the people with whom I stood in stunned disbelief, except that I would come back.

I was overwhelmed. I went to our branch office nearby where three of my colleagues were discussing the situation. I learned Darla hadn't been at home. She had been seen at a bar. Talk was it served her right to lose her kids. She deserved it, and so does the rest of Sunrise Circle. Talk was no more encouraging at the main office coffee break the next day. There was no recognition from my peers of how I might feel about having lost these five children. I repeated their names in my mind, Ethan, Lawrence, Denise, Unice, Nathan, over and over again.

The day of the fire it rained. I kept my appointment to moderate the dinner hour with the little girl and her retarded mom. When I came home after six o'clock, the daily newspaper, totally drenched from the rain, sat before the door with the headline story of the fire. I took it inside and cried into it as though it was the event itself. I also went out to buy a dry copy so I could read a version of what had happened.

Some facts are obscured, subject to opinion or interpretation. What happened was something like this. Around 2 a.m. the fire was spotted by a patrol car from the highway 3 blocks away and was called in. A Napier city fire station was directly next door to Sunrise Circle, but Sunrise Circle was in Elgin County, not Napier, so the station would not respond to the call. It took the county fire station a half hour to arrive on the scene. The fire probably began in a pot left on a back burner. It probably smoldered for quite awhile before becoming flames that were visible from the highway. The children were found in their beds and died of asphyxiation, not burns. Darla said she was sleeping on the couch and was awakened by the fire, running out of the house bare-foot. As the story unfolded in the news, the initial dispatch call was replayed frequently, sung to the tune of "London Bridge is falling down." It was twisted, instead, to the words of, "Sunrise Circle is burning down, burning down, burning down."

I never saw Darla again. She returned to the big city, where the funeral was held. The local churches hired a bus to take Sunrise Circle residents to the funeral. A worker from the department of aging, whom I had enlisted for Betsy's care, joined me in carrying a dinner to Betsy's home a few weeks later, when her other grandchildren were visiting. I called Darla at a number I was given. She called back. I said how sorry I was for her loss. I couldn't make anything right for her. She continued to be crucified by the public when talk turned to the Sunrise fire, although racism was noted by many in the refusal of the next door fire station to respond and the tone of the dispatcher's announcement.

Transformation was needed by the residents of Sunrise Circle, and many of the rest of us. The focus had to be on the children. Money was obtained for a summer recreation program. The county sponsored a special immunization clinic, which everyone attended. Parents examined their lives and moved on. I had an experience of driving to the airport 2 days after the fire on my way to a weekend in New York. I drove behind a taxi and suddenly noticed a baby waving at me, being held by his mother to wave at me, that is. Then I recognized that this was a Guatemalan mother and child whom I had also visited. They had survived the fire in their apartment building weeks before. I took it as a sign that the children don't always die. I still say their names though, Ethan, Lawrence, Denise, Unice, Nathan.

Sunrise Circle had become the epitome of everything bad in society: drugs, gangs, and prostitution. Scenes from Sunrise Circle replayed on the evening news in much the same way Rush Limbaugh plays background sounds of unruly crowds whenever he discusses "liberal" viewpoints. It is stereotyping of the worst order. Not only are individuals with their individual struggles not portrayed at all as themselves, but everyone associated with Sunrise Circle is guilty by association. In particular, they were guilty of attacking a representative of the system, the police officer, and not only the person or persons involved in the attack, but all of the residents of Sunrise, most of whom were children.

It is clear to me now that the baby scale I carried was roughly the same size as the grill used in the earlier altercation with police, a hard metal object that would not give in contact with human flesh. It symbolized my reason for being present on the "battlefield"—infants—but also constituted a defense for me personally.

Grandmother Betsy's home, where I met Darla, was organized and well kept. As I got to know Betsy, I became aware of her 18-year-old son, whose name I do not know. An 18-year-old living with parents is not unusual in the United States. But, as I now understand about families living in housing-funded communities ("The Projects"), it is necessary for the men to disappear and not exist so they do not jeopardize the family's welfare benefits. The only adult Black men I met in Sunrise Circle were pimps. They had enough power and control so they did not have to disappear.

I broke the rules by transporting Darla and the children to WIC clinic. WIC was co-located with public health nursing and county social service offices in a "one-stop-shopping" model that was supposed to facilitate access. Only it was in an industrial park that lacked public transportation. The rules did not hold universal sway for me. The future of the children did.

Darla reminded me of a Tracy Chapman song, "Fast Car," about the dream of moving beyond the constraints of poverty. Darla's attempts at wallpapering and buying fancy pink furniture on delayed credit fit the dream, but when she was on her own, things started to fall apart. Betsy wasn't a direct influence on Darla across the courtyard.

The fire and its aftermath were heartbreaking events. The memories of the residents were undoubtedly clouded by the rain, the dark of night and various conditions of drug or alcohol abuse. Among memories that may have been distorted was that Ethan called for help and that the firemen threw the bodies in the mud. I chose to believe the official account that the children never woke up, and that the fire fighters who did respond were respectful. The ongoing concern among the residents that emergency personnel would not respond to their calls for help was hard to refute.

Darla was never charged with neglect for leaving the children alone, the belief being that loss of five children was punishment enough. I held out another possible explanation for the children being left alone. It's possible that Darla left the children in the care of her brother, who was not supposed to exist because he was a Black male. Young Black girls learn very early to protect the boys, cover for them, and hide them. Darla's brother is the only member of the family whose name I didn't know, and this is significant to me; particularly considering that my continuous naming of the children was my attempt to affirm their personhood. Maybe it was Darla's brother who left the children alone, but Darla couldn't say that.

I felt a deep satisfaction in knowing individuals at Sunrise Circle and having the experience of relating to them in an intersubjective, I-Thou encounter. People responded to me, including the gang members who dispersed when I entered the project. Many individual encounters stand out in my mind. There was the home where I found 13 children and had to convince the adults that this was too many to be in one place at one time for daycare. It could have generated a call to the police or social services, but it was better just to work it out. Advising pimps on their everyday health concerns was a new experience for me.

We all grew as we moved through the motions of making Sunrise Circle a better place for children after the fire. It was like moving in slow motion amid the grief, but all of the adults took their places in the play, even some of the Black men who weren't supposed to be there and whose names I still don't know.

A place where nursing in the community thrives is called a nursing center. A nursing center is the hallmark of nursing in the community. It is a diamond in the rough, a pearl to be cherished in the inner city. These are settings that showcase the best in nursing coupled with the neediest in healthcare.

What is a nursing center? A spectacular place, a nurse-run clinic that is often affiliated with an academic institution where patients have direct access to nursing service (Barger, 2004). The focus is on diagnosing, treating, and promoting health or optimal functioning. The overall responsibility for the patient remains with the nurse. These settings are enormously successful because the nurse focuses on teaching and prevention. Underserved populations are targeted foremost (Fauchald, 2004). Typically, special populations of children, migrant workers, and refugees can receive care in a dignified healthful environment.

Stories from Agape Clinic follow. They are written by a family nurse practitioner, Charles Kemp. Agape is a community nurse-run clinic that uses a combination of medical and spiritual care, followup care for chronic disease, and community health services, while applying service-learning concepts in the clinic. The students of Baylor University School of Nursing are at the heart of this vision and perform outreach, case management, and home healthcare. The stories are dedicated to the volunteers from "La Clinica" who assist the nurses everyday.

BEING HUMBLED BY THE EXPERIENCE
by Charles Kemp (Texas, USA)

Last week was humbling. Actually, in this work most weeks are humbling—if we pay attention to who we are working with and what we are doing. First, there was a family from Chile. The wife was a university-educated midwife in Chile and is now working in a day care center. The husband was an executive financial analyst and is now driving a truck. Then there was a 5-year-old boy without parents in the home. He is cared for by his 18-year-old brother who is not doing too bad a job. Then there is the woman who brought in her feverish 4-year-old daughter. Her husband, an engineer, has been out of work for a year and has come to Dallas to go back to school. Several people in the family have been ill, and they spent all their money on the first three people who were sick. Further, we treated a 56-year-old dispossessed farmer from Zimbabwe. After losing his life's work he is starting over in America. There was a 2-year-old child with flaccidity, decreased intelligence and development, and the sweetest nature, and the most beautiful parents. And finally there was a 16-year-old who brought her grandmother to the clinic. The grandmother is from rural Mexico and is unable to read or write. Her granddaughter works with us as a Saturday volunteer and is planning on going to Baylor or Texas Woman's University to major in nursing. From generation to generation, country to country, hope to hope—how can we be so fortunate to do this work.

GETTING AT THE REAL ISSUES
by Charles Kemp (Texas, USA)

In the course of outreach, one of the students made several visits to an apartment where a 60-something-year-old woman lived with a younger man and woman. The younger woman was very reclusive, and every time we were there she had blood in her mouth (but no other evidence of trauma) and would not let us close enough to determine the problem. In conversations with the older woman, we learned that the man (call him Jimmy) was "helping" a 10-year-old girl who lived nearby. Over several weeks, the story came out that the girl had a bad home life. Her mother lived with two men and was intimate with both. The girl was afraid of one of the men and so spent as much time as she could with Jimmy. She bathed at his apartment, and at least once a week she spent the night with Jimmy, sleeping with him on a fold-out couch. According to the older woman, Jimmy and the girl liked to wrestle. Needless to say, when the story came out, we took quick action. I remember the student on this case saying in a very serious way, "Mr. Kemp, I think there may be a problem here." We talked with a detective of my acquaintance, and he went after Jimmy and brought Child Protective Services in on the case. I do not know the final outcome, except that the girl was removed from her mother's home and Jimmy disappeared. Good work, dear student.

HEALING IN NICARAGUA
by Anita Pursino (New York, USA)

It is sometimes said that people come into your life for a reason. I believe this to be true. I met Stu one day in October on a cardiac teaching day. Stu, a "Gringo Doc," talked to me about an upcoming VOSH (Volunteer Optometric Services to Humanity) mission. The timing and circumstances were perfect. It would be in January, a perfect time to escape the frigid winter temperatures in New York, and it would be a wonderful chance to meet new people and make new friends. Moreover, I had no urgent obligations.

This would be my first medical mission to Nicaragua. Friends and family thought me crazy due to the financial cost and the fact I spoke little Spanish, I knew little about the other people going and what was expected of me, and Central America was politically unstable at the time. I was asked, "Did you hear that a doctor was kidnapped just a few days ago in Bosnia? Do you really want to go?"

Had I really gone crazy? Did I really want to do it? I had a 15-year-old daughter who needed me. She was worried. What about helping underserved people and communities in the United States? After a week of soul searching and serious thinking, I made my decision. I heard a calling and saw a mission coming my way. I thought it was the right time and the right thing to do. I was determined to do it, and I would do it. People there need my help. I didn't know how, but I knew that God would help me figure out how.

On the day before my departure to Nicaragua, the gastoenterology associates offered me two cartons of cans of a supplemental "boost" drink; pediatric associates gave me about 10 cans of baby formula; and many doctors from Hyde Park gave me sample drugs to take along on the mission. All these contributions went into my carry-on backpack, which became heavier and heavier as I went from Poughkeepsie to LaGuardia Airport, to Miami Airport, and then on to Nicaragua. Heavy though my load was, I realized that it was worth more than all the gold and diamonds in the world when an emaciated 12-year-old girl, a 16-day-old failing newborn baby, and an elderly stroke patient benefited from these gifts. I began to understand what my mission was all about.

I managed to have my finger on every pulse of the activities of the mission. We set up our clinic in a public school in Monimbo, Nicaragua. You could find me assessing my patients, charting chief complaints, taking patient histories with the help of the translator, teaching patients in my broken Spanish, assisting in the minor surgeries, and changing dressings amidst the flies. I dispensed eyeglasses and medications; I pushed wheelchairs and strollers across the school yard; I chased a hypertensive dementia patient around the school yard while trying to check his blood pressure; I held a crying infant and comforted a frightened child while wishing that I could take them home instead of just giving them toys. I moved big boxes of supplies with the "boys," and I was the "bad" guy in crowd and mob control.

Picture our dental clinic, which wimps like me called the torture chamber. We had six chairs all lined up. They would be full of dental patients—mostly children—who were screaming, being held down, and/or trying desperately to escape while their rotted teeth were being pulled out. After a while, you just had to scream with them. Forget about what was taught in nursing school in America. With limited resources, time, and a great number of patients, we couldn't always follow the protocols of "confirm the procedure, explain it to the patient, make sure he or she understands the procedures and signs the consent for the procedure, assess the pain level and emotional support, give the patient instructions before the discharge, and follow up with a phone call the next day." All the patients received a stuffed toy and a few toothbrushes afterward. I don't know if they understood what we did or why we gave them "gifts" afterwards. I do know it made us feel better.

We also learned to be resourceful. We used Styrofoam cups to make spacers for children needing asthma medications but who had difficulty with the inhalers alone. We heard of a man who had treated his diabetes for 15 years by drinking his first urine of the day. I still smile when I think of the patient who asked if we could actually feel the worms moving inside his stomach during an abdominal examination. What an incredible experience! Naturally, you would find me working everywhere. No wonder I was called the "chameleon" nurse. I showed up everywhere!

I heard someone say, "VOSH, I'm all "Washed Out." How true it was! We were all stretched to our physical and mental limits. We took care of more than a thousand patients every day, and we worked for 4 days straight, 12-13 hours a day, with very few breaks. Sixty-five people were responsible for dispensing 2,021 prescription eyeglasses and sunglasses; performing 25 eye cataract surgeries; giving 2,276 eye, 1,628 medical, and 465 dental examinations—and we dispensed 41 wheelchairs, canes, and walkers. I was profoundly moved. Indeed, it was hard work, yet most of us can't wait to do it again.

None of us can forget the face of an 82-year-old farmer who wept with joy because cataract surgery helped him see again. And there was another farmer, with 33 grandchildren and 50 great-grandchildren, who had his right arm cut off in a robbery yet, amazingly, has a great attitude toward life—he is happy because he has fresh air to breathe.

I am thankful I was included in this mission. I have learned, and I have grown. I made friends for life. I, too, can see clearly. We did have some unexpected situations, including the breakdown of the bus delivering us from the airport to the hotel; the fact that there was no running water in the clinic; that two of our female missionaries were mugged and held at knifepoint; and that we missed a devastating El Salvadoran earthquake by 200 miles.

I am willing to risk it all to make a difference. This mission of vision will let the poverty-stricken people see what a beautiful world this could be. We all can have a vision and see that different skin colors can be brought together by a common calling. Together we all can make a difference … to make this world healthier, more beautiful, and more colorful.

It is the community nurse who is the instrument for the poor, help-less, elderly, and distraught. This is the nurse who needs thanks. Thank you for opening your eyes to a world that many do not see and do not care about. Thank you for responding with wisdom and fortitude to the social injustices our patients experience daily. Thank you for focusing on relationships beyond the hospital wards and medical jurisdiction. It is innovative nurses like Charles Kemp who care daily for those who are overlooked in healthcare. They are the behind-the-scenes heroes in healthcare. They make us proud.

This chapter is dedicated to all the community health nurses who contributed to this book and those who are the leaders and vision-aries in healthcare. I also dedicate this chapter to the nurses and vol-unteers of the Agape Clinic/Baylor School of Nursing who give so much of themselves, year-round and weekends, and who offer not only elixirs to heal the body, but medicine for the spirit. Their soul-fulness keeps our profession strong. This type of nursing is a ministry of serving, giving, and securing a pathway to peaceful and healthful restoration.

REFERENCES

Barger, S.E. (2004). Academic nursing centers: The road from the past, the bridge to the future. Journal of Nursing Education, 43(2), 60-66.

Drevdahl, D., Kneipp, S.M., Canales, M.K., & Dorcy, K.S. (2001). Reinvesting in social justice: A capital idea for public health nursing. ANS, 24(2), 19-32.

Fauchald, S.K. (2004). Using academic-community partnerships to improve healthcare services for underserved population. Journal of Multicultural Nursing and Health, 10(1), 51-58.

Leddy, S., & Pepper, J.M. (1998). Conceptual-Bases of Professional Nursing (4th Ed.). Philadelphia: Lippincott.

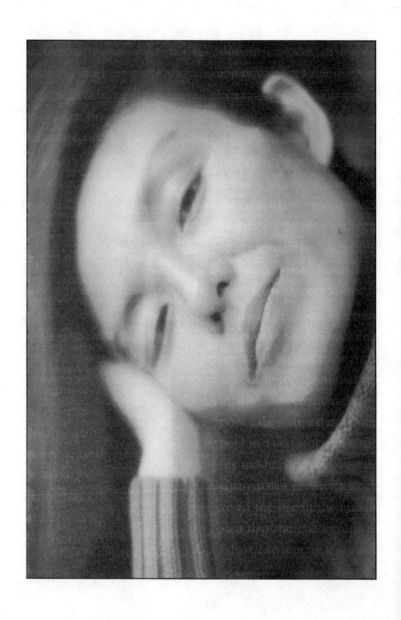

CHAPTER 6

Providing Comfort: The Ultimate Palliative Approach

These hands have helped heal and hold. So many patients, young and old, so many people, shy and bold, so many seasons, hot and cold. The touch of a nurse's hand is as precious as gold

—Jennifer McElligott Carley

Cancer. Death. These are the words that first come to mind when you hear "hospice." Leadership. Heroism. These are the words that describe hospice nurses. It is reassuring to know that these remarkable professionals are beside us when we need them, leading, loving, and heroically being. They create the bright light in the dark, giving the gift of consolation. They give people courage, grant a last wish, and take away pain with expeditious therapy. Whenever possible, they shape the final moments of life into a bundle of fulfilled memories.

Leadership. Lowney (2003) describes the secrets of leadership. He describes the four principles of leadership: understanding strengths, weaknesses, values, and worldviews; confidently innovating and adapting to a changing world; engaging others with a positive, loving attitude; energizing self and others through heroic ambitions. These main beliefs are followed by many nurses, particularly hospice nurses. They are inherent qualities used to assist patients at a time when there is little time. Hospice nurses make sure the patients' families are engaged, aware, educated, knowing about the disease and what is to come. They adapt to change; for example, they make it possible for a woman to die at home, in her own bed, overlooking what is important to her. They lead with love, because this work is the hardest and most challenging type of nursing.

Heroism. The word symbolizes nursing. It is the behind-the-scenes heroism that no one knows about, and that few outside of nursing value. The tremendous desire by nurses to keep their heroic work secret and sacred is puzzling, beautiful, and troubling all in one. Dr. Vassilik Lanara (1981) describes the bold, powerful work of nursing and states:"But above and beyond the intensive stress which characterizes every single nursing moment, what is unknown and incomprehensible to many is the heroism of the nurse's heart which day by

day, night by night, creates the unique meanings of nursing (p. 12)."
Do nurses want the memories to be known? Are they willing to rem-
inisce in the form of the stories they pen?

Hospice Nurses. Fast friends for humble people in need of comfort
and care. Hospice nurse are nurses who welcome people into the
innermost corners of their hearts. Hospice nurses are nurses who
assist on a journey.

What words are there to describe these incredible, giving, dedicat-
ed individuals? The hospice nurse is the person who sheds tears. The
hospice nurse is the person who respects the wishes of a woman who
wants to be photographed in a pink boa as her last memory. The hos-
pice nurse is the person who creates, for a family, its last Christmas—
in November—complete with a spruce tree, fine lights, and presents
strewn all over the hospital room.

It's hard watching a lump under the sheets, who was once a naval
officer, whither away. It is equally painful saying goodbye to a young
child. It is hard to grant one last wish, such as fresh air, overlooking
the pasture, being surrounded by loved ones, the scent of a burning
candle, holding one's wife close the night before death, but these
nurses make it happen.

Hospice nurses honor wishes, cherish dignity, lead in a system that
is afraid of death, by helping people die. Who wants to do it? Helping
families accept bad news—who would ever do this? Mature courage
and love is what it's all about. Courage, faith, strength, and love—
nurses report that these and many more attributes are the gifts they
get from patients and their families.

TAKING DIRECTIONS BY LISTENING
by Catherine Lopes (Florida, USA)

The day started like any other, with no significant moment to mark the beginning of a relationship that would affect me so deeply. I received report on a patient I would be taking care of, from another nurse who had a heavy caseload. She gave me the clinical picture of Frank. He was a 64-year-old man with a diagnosis of neck cancer. The surgery to remove the cancer had left a gaping hole in the right side of his neck, necessitating daily dressing changes. He was unable to swallow, had a feeding tube, and had also survived a carotid artery rupture. I was relatively new to hospice nursing, but I had a strong medical/surgical background and was very comfortable with my wound care skills. As I drove to Frank's home, I mentally rehearsed sterile technique, knowing it would be more of a challenge in the home setting than in the ordered environment of the hospital I was used to.

I rang the bell and heard a faint voice saying, "Come in." I was greeted at the door by Laddie, a timid Sheltie, and Brutus, a miniature Doberman with a very big attitude. They shuffled away as Frank entered the room. He was short in stature (5 feet 2 inches at the most), thin, and pale, yet carried himself with a commanding presence. I would later learn that Frank had been a career Navy man. A large bandage covered the right side of his neck, and his voice was raspy and difficult to hear. His demeanor was somewhat quiet. He was a man of few words. I let Frank know I would be his new primary nurse. I performed the assessment, did his wound care, and reviewed his medications. Everything was stable although Frank was not long for this world.

I visited with Frank on a daily basis, and I became close to him. He began to share his thoughts and concerns as I listened carefully to his raspy small voice. Frank had lost his wife of over 40 years during the previous year. She also had cancer, and he painfully described her decline. She had been a hospice patient for the last few days of her life and had in fact died at the local hospice house. Frank lived alone in the home they had shared. Knowing his prognosis was terminal, Frank was having repairs done to the house and had listed it with a real estate agent. He would silently slip to the neighbor's home when prospective buyers came. He searched for a home for his two pet dogs, and it broke my heart the first time I visited and was not greeted by the now familiar barking and tail wagging. Frank was a man who knew what had to be done and did it with bravery and courage.

Frank's two sons lived out of town and came to visit often. They were supportive of their father's decisions. I spent many quiet moments with them, explaining Frank's disease progression and what was to come and holding them when all the words were said. It is hard to watch grown men cry. They'd already lost their mother, now their father was dying.

As spring turned to summer, Frank's health continued to fail. By now we were close friends, and this quiet little man had made his way into my heart. We had our daily routine: taking his vital signs, completing an assessment and discussing ongoing symptom management and wound care. I would set up my supplies on his kitchen counter and bring in a chair for Frank. He would always thank me for the gentleness of my care. After we were finished, my reward was a hard candy from the jar on the counter. I always picked the blue ones.

Even with the tube feedings, Frank's nutritional and functional status continued to decline, and nausea sometimes broke through the antiemetics Frank took on a regular basis. We staggered our visits with his many friends so that Frank would not have to spend much time alone. He spoke periodically of stopping the tube feedings, for he knew that without it he would die sooner. I told him the facts and that I would support whatever decision he made. He decided to discuss it with his sons on their next visit and asked that the social worker and I be part of the discussion.

The five of us sat in the living room talking about how Frank would die without the tube feedings. The sons had already spoken with the oncologist who offered no further treatment options and a very realistic picture of Frank's condition. They did not want him to suffer, voiced their love for him, and vowed to live by his wishes. What awesome moments! A passerby would never have guessed what was being said in that tidy home with the neatly trimmed grass, the perfectly pruned flowers in bloom, the very picture of a safe and happy place.

Frank and I continued our daily visits. The amounts of his feeding fluctuated as he would cut back the amount, feel poorly, then decide to increase it again. I steadfastly remained in his corner, letting him make his own decisions, and kept the supply of nutritional supplements on hand. I changed his dressings and listened as Frank talked about how he wished for the end. There were no heroic moments, no machines to warn me of his impending death. The most important thing I ever did for Frank was to listen, really listen. He had few requests of me. Actually he had only one. Frank did not want to die at home. He didn't want his sons or his friends to watch him die. He wanted no death vigil. He wanted to die at the hospice house, as his wife had done. He knew I could not promise a bed would be available, but he trusted me to know when it was time. But would I know? This part of nursing was new to me and I feared I would miss the signs—after all, no machinery, no coworkers to catch the signs I might miss, no one down the hall to call on. I promised Frank I would do my very best and hoped that his trust was not misplaced.

In our many discussions, Frank related that he didn't want to go to the hospice too early. He wanted to be at home as long as possible, and he didn't want to be taking a bed from someone who might need it more than he did. I continued to listen and continued to gain knowledge of end-of-life care, and the signs and symptoms of impending death.

When the time came, I knew. I knew the rhythm of Frank, I recognized the obvious and the subtle, and I had been listening. I requested a bed for him, and I informed the sons. I listened and I silently prayed as the transport team was on its way.

The relief I felt at that moment was intense. I would never have forgiven myself if Frank had not gotten his one request. I went into the bedroom to tell him the news. He had gotten smaller somehow, barely a bump under the sheet. I sat there beside him and reached for his hand. Yes, there was a bed for him, but it also meant that this warm courageous man was soon to die. He looked me deeply in the eye; there was no place to hide. His eyes were so trusting as he asked, "It's time?"

"Yes, Frank, it's time," I told him. His son entered the room, and I slipped away to allow them some privacy. The transport van arrived, and I gently helped Frank onto the stretcher and followed him outside. Frank said that when he got to heaven he planned to be a guardian angel for all of the staff who had given him so much. I gave him a kiss and the professional wall fell away as our tears mingled on his small pale face. I never saw Frank again. He died less than 36 hours later, the epitome of dignity and self-directed care.

In this highly technologic time, listening has become somewhat of a vanishing art. Lab tests, MRIs, CT scans, and monitors are drowning out the patients' voices. We must try to continue to hear their voices above the din of the machinery. We must put down our clipboards long enough for them to know we are willing to listen to them—for their care should be self-directed, their priorities our priorities, their dignity self-defined.

The patient's last wish is the hallmark of caring. The patient needs to be guaranteed he will not have dreadful pain or shortness of breath. So many are afraid of "the death rattle." So many are frightened by the equipment. Nurses find themselves working so hard to do all they can to make the time spent at the end of life precious, for the patient and the family (Virani & Sofer, 2003). It may be just a little thing, such as a picture, religious ritual, or a room with a view of the sunset, flowers, and sweet smells. A last wish may be to be surrounded by family, a special dress, some special memory that will live on. It may be a college diploma, never received but valued tremendously. Whatever the request, it's never too big—or too small—for nurses who have great big hearts and the energy that could light up the world.

HONORING THE PATIENT'S WISHES
by JoAnn Slosek (Massachusetts, USA)

She wanted to die in front of her picture window, which looked out onto her lovely garden. It was late spring, and her flowers were all in splendid bloom. She had no relatives and had hired a private aid to take care of her. She was so sad and lonely. We managed to move her hospital bed to the window, and she died as she wished, looking out onto the wonderful garden that had become so important in her life.

COMPLETING A LIFE
by Cara Reed (Pennsylvania, USA)

Pills and intravenous (IV) fluids and other medical treatments are usually manufactured in large factories around the world. However, the greatest "medicine" I have ever given a patient—a resident—was actually created in an old country home in a small town called Laflin in the summer of 1981. Ever since I was a toddler, I loved to spend time with older adults like my grandparents and great-uncles and aunts. I was always comfortable around them, and I thrived on the unconditional love they gave me. My grandmother, Stella, played a very important part in my childhood. She taught me many "old-fashioned" things. I couldn't understand why I needed to learn to sew and cook, with all the modern conveniences. But, because I believed in the wisdom of elders, I learned all I could from my grandparents. One of the skills my grandmother handed down to me that summer of 1981 made a huge impact in one woman's life in the summer of 2003.

Catherine, a 99-year-old woman, lived at Mountain View for about 4 years. Each day, Catherine would spend hours at work creating beautiful baby afghans for her numerous grandchildren and great-grandchildren. She also crocheted lap robes for some of her friends at Mountain View. Her greatest joy was to give the gifts that she created with her hands. Catherine loved her hobby so much that she overcame pain from arthritis to continue to create her works of art. Time had caused Catherine to crochet at a slower pace, but not without the same beauty and personalization she added to each piece. Catherine was well-known throughout the Mountain View community for her crocheted works.

Even during times of acute illness, Catherine would get up each day and crochet. Her "workshop" in her room consisted of a small table, a gooseneck lamp, and a wicker basket that was always full of yarns of different colors. Catherine often chose to skip activities and events because she was busy with her work. Many grandchildren of Mountain View residents, as well as children of Mountain View employees, were wrapped in Catherine's "blankets of love" for their rides home from our long-term care facility. Catherine's life had meaning in that she shared her talent with so many others. I believed it was a beautiful intergenerational gift to wrap a newborn in something created by a 99-year-old.

In the summer of 2003, Catherine's terminal illness began to overcome her strength, and her body began to slow down. Through pain and frustration that she might not see her 100th birthday, Catherine continued to crochet until the last days before her death. She was on palliative care and required frequent doses of pain medication to keep her comfortable. Catherine's large family gathered around her bedside. They sat with her and spoke to her all the time she was alert. Catherine's dying process seemed unusually long, and it was almost as if she were fighting death.

As I usually did in situations like this, I asked the family members if she had been able to say her goodbyes to everyone. They told me that she had. Perhaps she was holding on for another reason. I asked them if she was afraid of death, but they agreed that she was looking forward to seeing her parents, husband, and young grandson in heaven. I continued with my questions by asking them if they had given her permission to go, but they had. Did she have some unfinished business, then? They looked to the wicker basket sitting on the floor next to her bed. It held an unfinished yellow baby blanket that Catherine had intended to give to one of the expectant nursing assistants.

I approached Catherine and spoke into her ear. I told her that I was not the best crocheter, but I would take the afghan home and finish it so that her daughters could give it to the baby it was intended for. Catherine gently smiled, a sure sign of her consent. Her daughter agreed that the afghan might have been what was keeping Catherine here. I took the 3 ft. by 1 ft. yellow yarn piece, which she had crocheted in her trademark popcorn stitch, along with the pink and blue yarn that she had picked out for the child. The afghan would be finished.

Catherine passed away peacefully that afternoon, just about 3 hours after she knew that her last task in life would be completed.

My grandmother, now 85 years old and a resident of Mountain View, gave me the very skill of crocheting in the summer of 1981. Now I know why she insisted that it was important, and that someday I would "need to know how to crochet." As a nurse, this was the best gift I have ever given someone. How ironic that the very woman who gave me the gift lived but 200 feet away from Catherine, and they never met. But through me, my grandmother helped to complete the circle of life for another grandmother.

The afghan was finished that weekend. After Catherine's burial, her daughters came to see the piece and cried in joy. They presented it to the pregnant woman and told her how special this blanket would be. Catherine was 99, my grandmother was 85, and I was 32; there were 216 years of love woven into that blanket. The baby was sure to be warm.

RECEIVING GIFTS FROM A DYING BOY
by Diana Peirce (Vermont, USA)

Daniel was born after what had seemed to be a normal third pregnancy for his mom, Janet. Like so many of us, Janet juggled home, care of children (4-year-old Jamie and 6-year-old BJ), work, and being a wife to Bill. When Daniel was born with severe birth defects, including multiple facial deformities, Janet was shocked and grieving, but there was never any doubt in her mind or heart about her love for this child. Daniel was transferred to a large medical center where specialists determined that he also had profound irreversible cardiac anomalies that would lead to his early death. "Two to four weeks life expectancy," was the verdict.

Janet told me of the day when the physicians suggested that the kindest thing to do was to withhold artificial nutrition from her weak, sick little boy, give him medication for comfort, and let him go. But, they didn't know Janet. It wasn't that Janet denied the terminal nature of her tiny son's condition. It wasn't that Janet minimized the difficulties inherent in caring for her little boy in spite of all the practical problems. It was simply that Janet had a great love for her child.

Daniel was transferred back to our local hospital leaving the specialists shaking their heads. Janet learned to administer tube feedings to Daniel to sustain his flickering life. It was at this time that I first met Janet and Bill and Daniel. Janet and Bill wanted to take Daniel home. I remember Janet telling me that she and Bill would do most of the care, but that they would need some support. If Daniel lived past Janet's 2-month leave from work, she would need more help providing care at home. Thus began our journey together.

Daniel lived at home for more than 3 months. During that time, he became an integral and important part of the family. We may never be capable of putting into words all of the lessons he taught us. Other than helping with his physical care, our task and our goal was to help this little family create a lifetime of memories in 3 short months—locks of silky red hair, little smiles, bright eyes turning to Mom's voice (even though Daniel was supposed to be hearing impaired), a family portrait—all were examples of the gifts Daniel gave us. Daniel's dad and little brothers had opportunities also, to hold him, to help feed him, to come to know him as the special little boy he was.

And when he died, I was privileged to share the moment. Family members gathered, and we took turns holding Daniel—it almost felt like everyone had a need to inter Daniel, not in a country cemetery, but in their hearts and spirits where he had held such an important place for several months. I will long remember the thoughtfulness of the funeral director as Janet handed the body of her little boy to him for gentle transit to his final rest. Yet, through the sorrow, I marveled at the courage, the gentleness, and the growth we had experienced, witnessed, and shared.

Yes, it probably would have been "easier" from a practical standpoint just to have let Daniel go. But Daniel had gifts to share—with his parents, his little brothers, and his hospice nurses. Gifts that we all shall treasure for a lifetime. Gifts that made Daniel's a meaningful life, and death.

MAKING A WISH COME TRUE
by JoAnn Slosek (Massachusetts, USA)

Phyllis was a hairdresser. She still dressed with a flare and always wanted to look perfect, even when she was too ill to even get out of bed. One day we were discussing what she wanted to accomplish prior to her death. She told me she would like to wear a pink boa and have her picture taken in front of her lilac bushes. She would then give a framed copy of this picture to each member of her family so they could remember her that way! The social worker and I bought the boa, dressed her up, put her in the wheelchair, and took her to the yard to take the picture. Her pure happiness showed in her face that day. Her family now had a wonderful remembrance.

CARING BY REACHING OTHERS
by Hayley Peterson (Missouri, USA)

I have never really had the desire to take care of people in nursing homes, and I was not looking forward to it. After my 2-week rotation at the home, however, I learned a lot about how a nursing home works and the type of care each patient receives, including interactions with nurses, doctors, and aides. I was able to see how I affected the life of one individual who was about to die due to serious complications of congestive heart failure and other disease processes.

When I was assigned to Joe, I was warned he was uncooperative and had a temper. I spent time giving him his medications, doing a full head-to-toe assessment, eating with him, talking with him, and helping him shower and change. Each day I discovered more about his personality and how he liked his day organized. Since he liked to get his medications early, I would locate the nurse to unlock the cart so he could take his medicines when he wanted. I think this made him feel more in control of his life.

While doing the assessment, I was able to find out about the pain he was having. I asked him about the location and the onset of the pain. I knew one of the main nursing priorities for Joe was pain management. I think it relieved his anxiety just talking about it. When Joe ate his breakfast, I would encourage him to eat all of his food so he would have adequate nutrition. I had seen the amount of food he had been eating and noticed it wasn't very much.

My favorite thing was hearing him talk about his family and his feelings. He would call his daughter occasionally and loved to talk about his grandson. He never wanted to go play bingo, so we would just sit and talk some more. I know our relationship was strengthened through this time because he started calling me "sweetheart" and always wanted to know when I was going to be there and for how long.

Valentine's Day was one of the days we were scheduled to go to the nursing home to take care of our patients. I made Joe a valentine, and he insisted I put it up on his TV so it blocked his view of the screen. It made me laugh, but I also felt special because that request told me he liked it and it meant something to him. Valentine's Day was also our last day together, so I told Joe I would no longer be coming to see him. I could tell he was sad about it. Joe and I had a friendship built upon trust. It took a listening ear and a little extra time in his room to develop this.

Joe's hospice nurse was also very nice and fun to know. She made jokes with Joe and asked me how he was doing. She stayed in the room and chatted with us, and Joe continued to smile throughout the entire visit.

Joe's hospice nurse was a friend to Joe. I was a friend to Joe. I believe these two meaningful relationships improved Joe's satisfaction concerning quality care. He ate more, which should have helped his nutritional status and homeostasis. I think he enjoyed being happy with good company more than he worried about his medications. I think talking with him about his family and his accomplishments in life helped him find closure and a sense of completion in his life.

LEARNING COURAGE, LOVE, AND COMMITMENT
by Diana Peirce (Vermont, USA)

I am a hospice nurse. Now, depending on your point of reference, such a statement may conjure up images of someone with a halo and wings ("Our hospice nurse helped us get through Dad's death."), or someone whose motivation you just don't understand ("How can you stand such a depressing job?"), or something in between. Regardless of the image, hospice nurses are most often thought of in terms of what we do or give. I would like to share with you some of what we receive, some of the gifts our patients give us.

For Charles and Pam, life was good. After years of hard work, they had built their "dream home"; their two children were grown and would soon marry. They looked forward to early retirement (both were in their mid-50s) and enjoying the fruits of their labor. Then, the unthinkable happened. Charles was diagnosed with lung cancer and given a life expectancy of less than 6 months. When I first met Charles and Pam, they were busy helping their two children prepare for their weddings—however, the dates were changed once Charles' condition was known so that he could be included. Charles could still walk at that time, and what a joy it was when he escorted his only daughter down the aisle to meet her groom!

Throughout the difficult late summer and fall, as the physicians' prediction of slow deterioration became fact, Charles' care became increasingly complicated. Bu Pam was always ready to meet the challenge. Through the anguish, when he could no longer walk and became confined to a wheelchair and then to a geriatric chair, through the indignity of losing bladder control, Pam's willing spirit, combined with Charles' sense of humor, kept them going.

Charles' goal that autumn was to live to dance at his son's wedding in mid-October. And dance he did. How proudly he displayed photos of himself dancing with his wife and with his new daughter-in-law, wheelchair and all!

One of the more difficult times came when Charles' respiratory status and care requirements dictated confinement to a hospital bed—which meant he and Pam were separated at night. But, in their usual fashion of making the best of a situation, Pam had the bed placed in the living room and decorated it and the walls around it. Frequently she slept in a recliner nearby, just to stay close.

When the holidays were upon them, Pam was determined to make the best of it, and Charles was determined "not to drag them down." Pam and the children set up and trimmed the Christmas tree next to his bed, a week early on December 5. Charles, who was bedridden and weak by this time, participated by "bossing the job." He lapsed into a coma on December 16 and died quietly with Pam at his side on December 18, one day after his 55th birthday.

Charles taught us to celebrate life, and he and Pam together gave us lessons in courage, love, and commitment. We grew stronger and more optimistic from knowing them.

GAINING NEW PERSPECTIVES FROM THE PATIENT
by Michelle C. Steinfeldt (Florida, USA)

She sat on the couch in her large bedroom, weak and small, but trying to be stoic in the presence of her adult children. Ms. D was the mother of five—three were mentally handicapped adults. All looked to me and the social worker, Ted, to "make it all better."

That was my introduction, that warm October day, to a lady who still had much to share.

Ms. D had experienced a rough night before we admitted her to our care. She had developed a salivary gland infection that only became symptomatic on her arrival home from the hospital, necessitating a return to the ER during the night, because she could no longer tolerate the pain. Oxycontin and antibiotics administered that morning had started to provide some relief. Nausea and constipation further complicated her rest as did extreme weakness, when she had to rely on one or two people to help her to the bathroom. With her consent, I ordered a walker, wheelchair, and bedside commode. She preferred to sleep in her own bed. I spent a few minutes instructing her family on walker use, standby assist with transfers, and ambulation as a means for providing some safety. Her three handicapped children, B, L, and J, were high functioning microcephalics, and they eagerly listened to instructions and told me proudly, "We can take good care of Mom while A is at work." A was gone from 8 to 5, so Ms. D relied on them for meals, housekeeping, and help in A's absence. Another son, R, was expected to take a leave from his job in Chicago and move in. Ms. D was confident this plan would work.

Three days later, she was obviously more comfortable, and the mandibular swelling had receded due to the medications. She was able to keep an accurate log of her pain and asked A and R to review the log and the results of the scans and other diagnostic tests conducted at the hospital. Using pictures of the chest and abdomen, I described Ms. D's condition. We talked about how cancer metastasizes and how the pancreatitis created the need for hospitalization when the cancer was detected initially with a chest film 2 weeks before. She listened quietly and then turned to her son saying, "I just want to be comfortable." In a weak, but assertive voice, she turned to me and said, "Can you folks help us in securing guardianship of the three younger kids by the boys? They have always been together and A and R have agreed they will take care of them when I'm gone." I informed her I would ask Ted, the social worker, to contact them. He would know the best way to advise her. We talked about the younger kids and how they would react with her decline. I promised to talk with them each visit—it was easy to recognize their need to be involved in "Mom's care." Praise and recognition of their efforts helped to develop trust and certainly promoted their comfort with our staff's presence in the home. At each visit all three of them met me at the door, eagerly telling me what each had done for Mom. They brightened with smiles when I praised their accomplishments.

L, the only daughter, was especially good at anticipating her mother's needs and spoke with pride about her nursing care. Ms. D, alone, managed her medications, but admitted she had a poor memory and transient confusion, which she blamed on the medications. She agreed to my setting up a medication box for each day and was further relieved when I told her I would continue to fill them for her. I was particularly struck by her openness and determined self-care in the face of a progressive disease. I was eager to support this, and each visit I was rewarded with her living example of human grace in the face of adversity and impending death.

By early November, Ms. D was showing signs of disease progression with increased pain through her chest and into her back and abdomen. She had bibasilar crackles but continued to deny dyspnea. Her upper abdomen was firm, and a palpable mass was easily felt one handbreadth below the left ribcage—it was tender to the touch. After conferring with the pharmacist, we adjusted her pain medication. Further assessments of Ms. D determined new comfort measures and methods were needed to promote what little appetite she had.

With each successive visit, I could see the concern in the eyes of the younger kids. Her daughter recognized Ms. D's changes and one day broke into tears. "Mom's sicker, isn't she?" We talked about the medicine helping to control pain and nausea, and I supported her awareness of her mother's decline while praising all she was doing to promote her comfort. She knew just what foods to fix and kept her mother's water fresh. When alone, Ms. D and I talked about her increasing weakness, anorexia, and jaundice. I taught her about disease progression, reminded her we would continue to adjust her medications, and shared my concern for her safety during the day while A was at work. She told me her other son, R, would arrive that weekend.

November 21 brought another increase in pain medications for unrelieved pain in her upper back and abdomen. She was sleeping more and eating less and her bowel function had slowed. Coarse crackles were heard in the mid/lower lobes of both lungs now, and she had difficulty breathing with any exertion. We added medication for probable bone pain, although Ms. D couldn't differentiate organ from bone pain. Oxygen was ordered, and I spent considerable time with her son, R, teaching him about his mom's expected disease progression, care giving techniques, and ways to record pain. After telling me he was shocked to see her so sick, he admitted with tears in his eyes, "I thought I could come down here and help to get her better—she's really dying, isn't she?" I listened while he talked about his 4-year absence from Florida. His last visit was when his father died suddenly of a heart attack at home. His 19-year-old son was with him this trip and listened intently to our conversation. R had already identified the need for his siblings to be prepared for Ms. D's death and asked many questions about when, how, and what to do as his mom's time grew shorter. He would continue to involve them with A and help them to understand what was coming. I saw in R the gentle supportive side that A didn't show, and together, they kept the household running smoothly as their mother continued to decline. At one visit, their difference was particularly evident. A was replacing a defective water heater while R saw to Mom's breakfast and medications, but both sought direction and encouragement for what they were doing for her comfort.

After Thanksgiving, the older sons had completed the guardianship legalities and realized there was a need to make funeral plans. After discussing with Ms. D what she wished to do, R visited the local funeral director. "It was the hardest thing I have ever had to do," he reported. I saw in his eyes the grim reality of what was ahead, but he voiced relief at finding out what Ms. D wanted.

When I visited on November 27, Ms. D had been seen by one of our night nurses after she developed difficulty swallowing. Thrush was identified and Nystatin ordered. As I entered her room, she smiled and through a groggy weakness said, "What's next?" She requested a urinary catheter, saying, "I'm too weak to get out of bed." R and his sister took this all in stride and reassured Ms. D they could manage the care of a catheter. With another increase in pain medication, Ms. D spent most of her days sleeping. It took careful questioning to determine her pain levels. R kept her medicated for comfort. His dedication to her comfort reinforced my awareness of the loving relationship of mother and son.

When I called the next day, R noted Ms. D's unresponsiveness and transient periods of no breathing. She had declined oxygen, saying, "It doesn't help." His observations proved true, and my teaching focused on continued preparation of the family for her death. The younger kids seemed more anxious but asked few questions. I had to seek them out to offer support. All three could only say, "Mom's real sick, we know, R and A told us." L walked from the room crying and refused to be comforted. R noted L had become quieter and often sat at her mom's bedside holding her hand while she slept. I reinforced this as a positive sign of her coping and urged him to continue to encourage her to do this.

On November 30, R informed me Ms. D was gurgling. We administered new drugs to ease her difficult breathing. As I was leaving the home, the family seemed subdued but asked if there was anything more to be done for Ms. D's comfort. I reinforced hand holding, prayers with her if she desired them, and for each one of them to tell her it was OK to go when she was ready. Our agency chaplain made a visit, also. R reassured me, "We'll be OK till Monday—I'll call if needed." He reminded me he had read the "Final Days" section in our handbook and knew what to watch for.

Ms. D died peacefully in the presence of her sons, R and A, at 4:00 a.m. on December 3. They chose not to wake the three younger children or her grandson. I visited the family later the same day to find them grieving appropriately. B and J told me they had said goodbye before they went to bed the night before but were surprised to see her gone in the morning. A graveside service for Ms. D was planned. Each of the family members spoke easily with me but L withdrew to her room. I praised the loving care each had provided. They commented that "now Mom is at peace and no longer hurting" and suggested I not try to talk to their sister now. R and A reiterated they would be able to manage guardianship and the home.

In my many years of nursing, I've cared for many different families and patients. Ms. D and her family have made a particular impression on me, deep in my soul, and one I shall not soon forget. Her acceptance of her diagnosis and openness in allowing outsiders to share her final walk truly showed her grace and spirit. Strong yet vulnerable, confident and trusting, she gave her children and those of us who knew her a role model. I look back now and realize that while ministering to my patient and her family, I was also receiving the benefits of her life well lived, and an example of humanity at its best. She was indeed a very special person.

DOING THE IMPOSSIBLE
by Debra N. Fisher (New Jersey, USA)

To begin, I am a hospice nurse who cares for people in their homes. The area I serve is a very rural area of New Jersey. All of the nurses in our agency take turns accepting weekend "on-call" time. Typically we end up with at least two different weekends of "on-call." Usually this time consists of more than 24 hours at a time, after working the week. Our on-call includes checking on people any time, day or night. As nurses, we strongly encourage our families to call with a problem. It's more important to call—even if it's two o'clock in the morning—than to ruminate and worry all night. After all families have been through, they need the reassurance of knowing there is someone out there who can help at any time.

One night I was on-call. I got a phone call from a man whose wife was one of our patients. The woman had metastatic lung cancer. I was not a primary nurse for this patient; in fact, this was the first time I had ever spoken to them. The woman's name was Lucy, and her husband was Jim. Lucy was rarely able to swallow without choking, due to disease progression and the treatment that was provided. Lucy had a tube that was used to provide food for sustenance. Unfortunately she continued to drain oral secretions, which would cause her to choke occasionally. Some medications seemed to be helping dry some of the secretions. Her primary nurse had a suction machine delivered that Lucy could use independently. This was very helpful and reassuring to both Lucy and Jim.

I received a call about 1:30 a.m. on a Saturday morning with news that the suction machine wasn't working. They tried to get it working, but their efforts were futile. I told them I would be there as quickly as I could.

When I got there, I found I was out in the middle of nowhere. It was really dark, except for the lights in the house itself. The driveway was long and a distance from the house. I had to walk a long path over large uneven stones to get to the house. Lucy and Jim both looked exhausted. They could barely keep their eyes open. At times Lucy would make horrible gurgling sounds and get a terrified look in her eyes.

I tried everything I could think of to get that suction machine to work, but to no avail. I dialed the emergency number of the company who made the equipment and got an answering service. They said they would page the person on-call and get back to me in a few minutes. We waited and waited; after 30 minutes I called back. The answering service told me no one had called back yet. I explained the seriousness of the situation. Again I was told we would get a call back soon.

In the meantime, Lucy was getting more anxious and short of breath. I gave her medications to ease her anxiety and respiratory distress. We waited another half-hour, and still no call back. I was getting angry, but I knew it was important to be as upbeat and calm as possible.

I started to mentally review my options. It really didn't seem the equipment company was going to be helpful. I called the hospital and asked if the nursing supervisor could be paged so I could talk to her. After a few minutes, the nursing supervisor got on the line. I explained the entire situation. I explained how much more comfortable Lucy would be with a functioning suction machine. I asked if it was possible to borrow a hospital suction machine. She said, "Of course you can borrow a suction machine, don't ever hesitate to call us, I'll have the suction machine waiting for you in the emergency department. You will need someone to help you; it is heavy." I thanked her profusely. It was such a good feeling to get that kind of reaction and help. Lucy and Jim overheard the conversation and looked so relieved. I told them to be patient because it would take me a while. I would return as quickly as I could.

I drove the 18 miles to the hospital, in the dark, frequently passing deer on the roadsides. As I walked into the ED I saw the suction machine. It was fairly large, but it was on wheels. It was difficult to get into my station wagon, but I did, eventually. I raced back to the house, through the dark. After pulling the suction machine out of the car, I gingerly wheeled it over the long, uneven stone path. When I got to the house, there was no one downstairs. No one heard me arrive, and I didn't want to startle anyone. I dragged that thing through the house. Then I carried it up the steep steps. It was heavier than it looked. When I got to the top of the steps, Jim grabbed it. He said, "I can't believe you didn't call me. I thought I heard someone so I came to see what it was. What is that thing? It looks like you brought us a barbecue. It looks heavy and cumbersome."

We set the suction machine up in their bedroom and turned it on. It worked beautifully. Both of them looked so relieved. I left and got a little bit of sleep. I called Lucy and Jim later that day. They said everything was fine. The suction machine was working well.

Afterword, reviewing this event at my team meeting, the group all thought it funny. The primary care nurse had talked to Lucy and Jim. They had joked about me bringing the barbecue. They also were very thankful for my help. I felt such a relief to know that at one moment there was an unsolvable problem and the next it was resolved.

End-of-life care is managed by nurses who are able to solve many problems and overcome barriers every day. Even though the problems and barriers are beyond their control, they use all the resources available at the moment to solve the problems, make the patient more comfortable, and carry on. Faulty equipment, poor service from home care equipment companies, disorganization, and financial reimbursement issues are just a few of the situations they must address. The Institute of Medicine has identified four problems in end-of-life care: the overuse of care or unwanted treatment; the under use of care such as late referral to hospice; poor technical performance such as mismanaged pain; and inept communication of what is really going on with the patient (IOM, 1997). Nurses realize and live these shortfalls, guarding against inappropriate aggressive care, collaborating with social workers to minimize financial burdens, helping the family with bereavement, and ensuring a peaceful death.

Nurses sometimes have the really hard job of helping patients plan the final days. Assisting with funeral arrangements or selecting Scripture readings with patients is part of what they do. Many want, in advance, to plan their final moments and even those after. It is the nurse who is often the only one there who can help the patient read the Bible or plan a religious ritual. The patient doesn't want the family to know or worry.

GIVING MEANING TO THE END-OF-LIFE JOURNEY
by Mary K. Brodeur (Florida, USA)

Mrs. L was an older woman who had been diagnosed with ovarian cancer some time ago and was in the advanced stages of the disease. Her husband was very supportive. He brought her to each of our support group meetings and sat in the hallway or out in his car during the meeting. Mrs. L was a very proud woman and, despite this debilitating illness, tried her best to carry herself as straight and tall as possible. She was aware of, but undaunted by, the fact that due to treatment of her disease she had gained weight, lost her once-beautiful hair, and was unable to knit and crochet with the dexterity she once possessed. She told me even cooking and cleaning, which I probably considered a necessary dredge (and she was correct), were things she longed to be able to do again. She especially wanted to be able to cook and serve her husband a meal, but this was one goal Mrs. L would never again attain.

On one of my visits to Mrs. L while she was still at home and after her priest had started visiting, she surprised me by asking if I would bring a Bible the next time I came so we could look up some of the Scriptures she used to read. I did this, and we spent several hours finding the ones she loved and read them over and over together. After some time, she told me she would like to choose the Scripture readings for her funeral and asked if I would help her plan the services. I told her I would be honored to help her in such a personal and special way. After we chose Scriptures and songs and organized the service, she took a piece of paper, yellowed with age, from within the pages of a book that was always on the table at her side. She handed me a poem, asked me to read it then and at her funeral. She said it spoke to her about what the end of this journey of life was about. I would like to share the poem with you now.

I am standing on the shore.
A ship spreads its sails to the morning breeze
And starts for the ocean.
I stand watching her until she fades on the horizon,
And someone at my side says, "She is gone!"
Gone where?
The loss of sight is in me, not her.
Just at the moment when someone says,
"She is gone," there are others watching her coming.
Other voices take up the glad shout,
Here she comes!
That is dying.

I feel I made a difference in the final months and days of the life of Mrs. L. I know she made a difference in my life forever!

BREAKING THE RULES WHEN NECESSARY
by Kristina Cornell (Michigan, USA)

I had been working as a pediatric nurse for about 4 years, and nothing I was taught in school or learned on the job could have prepared me for what I went through in April of 2002.

The unit where I worked had a wide variety of patients and illnesses; unfortunately these included oncology patients. It is very difficult to see parents bring their children in for what they thought were childhood complaints, such as common aches and pains, bruises, etc., and within 24 hours, watch as their lives are turned upside-down when they are told their child has cancer. It is very hard to console parents during this initial period of adjustment as they are usually going through different emotions such as denial and anger. It is also very difficult to know what to say in these situations. Sometimes silence is what they need. People deal with this sort of adjustment in their lives in many different ways.

In the summer of 2001, a very bright, talented, outgoing 16-year-old boy named Javon was admitted to the hospital for complaints of right shoulder pain. This was a very fit, athletic boy, so we really didn't think much of it. A series of routine tests, such as x-rays, blood work, etc., were performed, and within a day or two, he was diagnosed with acute myelogenic leukemia (AML). The oncology team spent quite some time with him and his family explaining the disease and the possible treatment options. I was the nurse taking care of Javon the night he was diagnosed, and for the next few days. I did the best I could to comfort them and answer any questions I could; they had none. His family left for the night. I found it rather odd that his mother was showing no signs of grief. She didn't cry—didn't really react at all. Neither did Javon. I assumed they were probably in denial, which is a very common phase we see parents go through in these situations. But this behavior seemed to continue. I would constantly try to keep the family updated on everything I could, such as test results and lab results. I also gave them encouragement, trust, whatever I could. While they seemed to appreciate it, they rarely asked for anything.

Javon's father was not involved in his life, but the mother appeared to be a loving mother. She was very friendly and caring, but she did not seem to be concerned with her son's new diagnosis, nor did she seem to realize how serious it was. The days passed, more tests were done, and Javon was started on a chemotherapy regimen. In the next several months, we nurses became very close to him. He would be in and out of the hospital for either his scheduled chemotherapy treatment or with fevers/neutrophenia (low white blood count). In the latter case he would need to be put into isolation for his own protection. The family never stayed with him. He frequently had groups of friends visit him, as he was a very popular 10th grader. He was always in the best of spirits, walking around the unit, pushing his IV pole with one hand and holding his pants up with the other. His jeans always appeared to be four sizes too large, but this was apparently the style. I used to tease him about them and tell him I was going to buy him a belt one day, and he would just laugh and say that he had one in his room. It always amazed me that no matter how sick he was or how awful he felt, he never complained, even with all the 6:00 a.m. blood draws or the medi port checks in the middle of the night. He never got annoyed or irritated. At least he never showed it. He never lost his high spirits. Everyone enjoyed his presence.

Our oncology patients all get a "wish" from the Make-A-Wish Foundation, something that they want to do or see badly and would otherwise never get a chance to do. Some choose a trip to Hawaii, or meeting their favorite celebrity. Javon picked a trip to Disney World. Just a month or so before he was to leave, he cancelled it. He said his wish was to get a job and buy a car so that he could help his mom, who was a single mother with younger children at home and a limited income. He just didn't want his mom to have to struggle. This selfless act on the part of a 16-year-old boy amazed us, though it fit him perfectly. He never did get a chance to get a job or a car since his admissions to the hospital became more frequent and his immune system weaker. On his last admission, the end of March of 2002, he was transferred into the pediatric intensive care unit (PICU) because of extremely high temperatures, hypotension, tachycardia, and the fear of septic shock. We were all concerned but kept our fingers crossed in the hopes that all the high-dose antibiotics and constant one-on-one monitoring would eventually send him back to our unit. I would constantly inquire about his condition. A PICU nurse told me he was getting narcotics on top of the morphine PCA he was receiving and that a few times he yelled at her about needing more pain medicine. I was shocked to hear that he was being demanding, this was just not him, but I kept telling myself he was hurting and no one took it personally. I later learned that he had apologized to the nurses for yelling at them. In the midst of all this extreme pain, he still was polite and concerned about others and how they felt. This was the Javon I knew. Within a week, he was transferred back to the pediatric unit. We were all thrilled he had overcome the problems that had put him in the PICU, but it was really just the opposite. The antibiotics had fought the infection enough to stabilize his temperature and blood pressure, but he had contracted a form of pneumonia called pneumocystis carinii. We were also told he was going into congestive heart failure (CHF). The oncology doctors basically told Mom there was nothing else they could do for him at this point, and he was transferred to hospice care.

When he was brought back to our unit, he was not the same 16-year-old boy I remembered. He appeared old. He was very weak and about 10 pounds heavier due to severe water retention. He was on oxygen and was not able to talk for very long before becoming short of breath. Per the family's request, he was kept on our unit for hospice care instead of going home, which is where hospice usually takes place. We were to provide comfort care only. His mom was concerned about his siblings at home (pre-school age) seeing their older brother like this. She also said he felt close to the pediatric staff, and she wanted him out on our floor where he felt comfortable, as opposed to the PICU.

The next 4 days were the most emotionally draining 4 days of my career as a nurse. We have a very strict policy regarding visiting hours and the number of visitors a patient can have at one time, but we made an exception in this situation. Over the next 4 days, there were at least 20 visitors at any given time, sleeping in the hallway outside Javon's room, in his room, and in the parent lounge. These crowds were in contrast to the few family members who were there earlier. It was amazing how close this family really was and how many people loved him. I would pay my visits and give him a hug, although by this time he didn't really recognize anyone. We watched him go from a cheerful, pleasant 16-year-old boy full of life, to someone who had the appearance of a 60-year-old man in a matter of a week. Every day I left work in tears. We all prayed for Javon and for his family, but on April 12 Javon passed away sitting in his recliner chair. The next few hours were amazing to me. After the family was able to say their goodbyes, we told them we had to get him into bed and get him cleaned up to take him downstairs to the morgue. Several of his uncles insisted on helping us and after several attempts of trying to persuade them to let us do it, we thought this was probably a way for them to gain closure and we couldn't deny them that. His uncles picked him up out of the chair and carried him in his bed. When all was done, his family thanked us immensely for allowing them to have that closure.

Several times a month, I think of Javon and how strong he was at just 16 years old and how he always put others' feelings ahead of his own, no matter what. Every time I think of him, it makes me smile. Life is too short. I will never forget him.

The holidays for many patients and their families are particularly difficult. All the past memories come flooding by. The smells of cinnamon, balsam fir, and holly berry become a sad memory. Celebration is hard if not impossible.

Many people are in hospice care around the holidays. The nurses are there for them and for their families, making special moments happen even if resources are scarce and the spirit of the holiday dampened. Nurses bake Christmas cookies for patients, buy gifts, even plan Christmas early so the family can have one last time together. Nurses don't take Christmas or Christmas Eve off. They leave their families to be with someone else's family.

Ask any nurse if she or he has worked on Christmas Eve. They all have. Ask any nurse if she or he has a special memory about the time spent with patients on Christmas… They all have.

It is always hard for hospice nurses to be away from their own families and friends on holidays, but as you read the next few stories, some of the greatest moments for nurses have, in fact, occurred on a day when most of the world is home by a fire celebrating with loved ones.

SHOWING DEDICATION
by JoAnn Slosek (Massachusetts, USA)

Tim had a 2-year-old son. Tim was not doing well in November, and during a conversation said, "If I had one wish before I die, it would be to see my son enjoying his second Christmas." I gathered my team together, and we decided to have Christmas in November that year. It was unbelievable to me the dedication the team showed. A volunteer went out and cut down a Christmas tree. He bought a stand, went to the house, and set up and decorated the tree in one afternoon. The home health aids all got together and baked Christmas cookies. The nurses went shopping, not only for the son, but also for the patient's wife and stepdaughter. Even the clerical staff were getting into the spirit. Gift certificates were piling up on my desk! Tim had jokingly asked us to buy red lingerie for his wife, and our social worker bought them, wrapped them, and put the box under the tree. The pastoral counselor dressed up as Santa and gave out the gifts. It was a sight to behold. Tim cried when he was presented with the gift of Christmas. Through our tears, we watched as this family enjoyed their last Christmas together.

Tim's wife actually stayed with him in his hospital bed that night. She insisted that the red lingerie be buried with him, and it was.

Granting the last wish, calming fears, assisting patients' transitions to peace—these are just some of the influences of the hospice nurse. They pay their final respects to the patient in the words they have written. They treasure these memories like a box of jewels never opened. For many, they have never told these stories. They have given them to us to read and appreciate. They have protected these words. Now, with devotion, they release the memories to us, for us.

Gratitude is extended to hospice nurses who every day appreciate the goodness in life and the inevitability of death, to nurses who fight their way through a tangled system of healthcare to honor their patients' final requests. We worship their work. We thank every hospice nurse for the love, respect, and dignity provided in end-of-life care.

REFERENCES

Institute of Medicine. (1997). Accountability and quality in end-of-life care. In, Approaching death; improving care at the end of life. Washington, DC: National Academy Press.

Lanara, V. (1981). Heroism as a nursing value: A philosophical perspective. Athens, Greece: Sisterhood Evniki.

Lowney, C. (2003). Heroic leadership. Chicago: Loyola Press.

Virani, R., & Sofer, D. (2003). Improving the quality of end-of-life care. Making changes at every level. AJN, 103(5), 52-60.

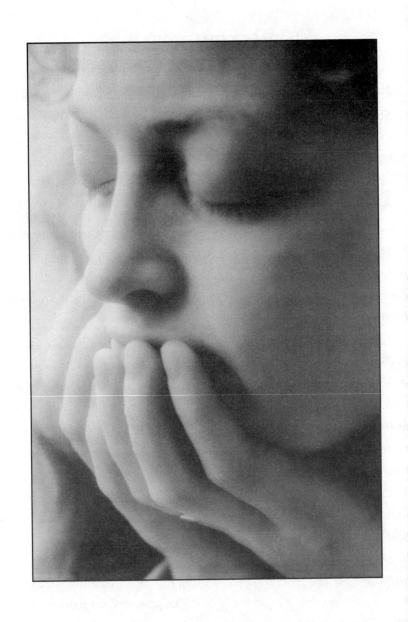

Chapter 7

Initiating Crisis Interventions

The sound of sirens, the smell of smoke, flashing lights, and chaos, police cars everywhere, a screaming mother, shock and disbelief, severed limbs lying about, gunshot wounds, gang fights: These are some hallmarks of a crisis.

Experienced, quick-thinking emergency department (ED) nurses expect the unexpected. They never know what will come through the door. Their education serves them well as they rapidly assess physiologic parameters. The hours spent in advanced critical-care training, testing, and continuous competency checks keep these women and men prepared. This is not a 9-to-5 job. It includes shift work, holiday work, and weekend work.

Nurses are prepared to respond to a range of emergencies that are relatively new to nursing. These include bioterrorism attacks with a host of biological agents: anthrax, smallpox, tularemia, and viral hemorrhagic fevers (e.g., Ebola virus). The complexity of emergency nursing since the 9/11 terrorist attacks on the United States has put a new spin on the role of the nurse. These healthcare workers must know how to recognize pruritic macules and the symptomatology of smallpox and anthrax and be able to isolate patients with great rapidity. In addition, "decontamination" is now an ED household term.

Nurses never know if they are targets, or if they will be pushed, punched, or bitten. The ED is not an environment for novices or for the weak at heart. Excrement, blood, spit, lice, and used needles are everywhere. It is not a pretty setting. Who knows what even the most seemingly mild-mannered patient might do?

ED nurses must also know how to protect children. Traumatic emergency events often include children directly or indirectly. The impact of stress on children must be recognized and managed. It is vital for nurses to use all the support systems available to help children manage crisis anxiety and grief. Involving family, teachers, coaches, and other significant adults is essential (Davidhizar & Shearer, 2002).

The stories drawn from the experiences of ED nurses are a powerful testament to their practice. The memories of special patients and families are close at hand. From the entrance of the ED to the swooshing doors in the ICU, critical-care nurses stand by. They are there for you and me, our families, and our loved ones, just in case a crisis comes our way.

CONTINUED VIGILANCE
by Erika Kelly Hinson (Florida, USA)

I admitted a restless Mr. B into emergency department room #14. He was very sweaty, clammy, and quite pale. He was oriented to person, place, and time, and he was complaining of chest pain radiating to his upper back and neck. Any deep breath or movement caused the pain to worsen.

My assessment indicated Mr. B had clear lungs, a 100% paced rhythm at 82, and soft abdomen with good bowel sounds and no tenderness. His blood pressure was 104/60, and his pulmonary parameters were normal. He had a history of cardiac changes in the past with insertion of a pacemaker 1 week earlier. He also suffered from hypertension and gastric reflux. He was recently widowed and had a son who lived in another state.

Suddenly, he complained of feeling dizzy. His skin was clammy, and he was very pale. His blood pressure had dropped to 72/43, his pulse was 82, and his respirations were 22. I lowered his head, turned off the nitro (a drug used to open heart arteries), and opened wide a normal saline fluid bolus with additional fluids. Moments later, his blood pressure was back up, his pain had lessened, and he was less clammy. While in an upright position for a chest x-ray, he complained of crushing chest pain at 10 on a scale of 1-10 and had again turned gray and pasty.

I asked Mr. B to lie flat, which reduced his pain to a 2 and restored his blood pressure and color. Numerous tests were conducted to evaluate his condition, and I accompanied him during the tests to monitor his volatile condition and provide reassurance.

I noticed he was continually moving his shoulders back and forth in bed and was restless. No amount of pillow fluffing or positioning helped him get comfortable. He was very concerned about letting his son know he was in the hospital. I called his son, and Mr. B seemed more relaxed. His vital signs stabilized, and I thought he might rest. I noticed his skin was dry and cool; however, he was frowning even with his eyes closed. He seemed very worried. He said he thought he had had a stroke. I reassured him that his neurological status was intact.

The extensive tests all came back with normal results, and the ED team considered discharging him. The doctor who was working in the

ED left for the day. Mr. B was not assigned to another ED physician because he was considered ready for discharge. When I elevated the head of his bed slightly, his pain returned to a 10 and his blood pressure dropped to 80/40, despite having had two liters of saline. I thought he had a serious problem. I realized I could not prove this man was sick, but my nursing instincts and intuition, as well as my professional experience in critical care, set off an alarm. When I had Mr. B lie down, his pain was alleviated and his blood pressure improved—two important parameters!

I called Dr. Y, knowing it would be difficult to get him to admit Mr. B, yet I felt compelled to do so. I related my concerns and asked for admission orders, only to hear him angrily say that he and the ED doctor discussed discharge. Again, I explained that Dr. X was gone, and I felt this man was acutely ill. After protesting, Dr. Y agreed to evaluate Mr. B when he finished his current patient's procedure. While waiting, Mr. B's pain returned to 9, even lying flat. His blood pressure went down, and he again was clammy. Soon, Dr. Y examined Mr. B and felt that, indeed, he might have pericarditis and should be admitted.

Continuing his evaluation, Dr. Y sat Mr. B upright, which resulted in crushing chest pain, dizziness, and vomiting. Dr. Y instructed me to get the cardiac catheter team on call. At last Mr. B had a diagnosis: acute pericardial tamponade with hypotension, secondary to pericardial effusion, presumed secondary to lead perforation status post-pacemaker insertion. Mr. B went to the ICU. When my shift ended, I knew my perseverance and concern had made a major difference.

Normally, we get almost no follow-up on our admitted patients, but a few days later, my director received a letter from Dr. Y. It said: "I would like to commend her on her astute findings and persistence in describing to me how ill one of my recently admitted patients was … I think she should be commended in reference to her caring nature of this patient and her continued vigilance and wary eye. These problems can be difficult to diagnose ... I would like to thank her personally for rendering "critical" nursing to a patient who needed it most."

PAYING ATTENTION TO INTUITION
by Anita Pursino (New York, USA)

When I went into work that day, I did not plan on saving someone's life. I had just started to receive the first patient's report when an attending neurologist arrived to examine another patient with a diagnosis of seizures. The physician wanted to do a spinal tap.

The neurologist had examined the patient and ordered an electrocardiogram (EKG) because the patient had experienced a seizure the night before. He was seen by the emergency department (ED) physician and was sent home and told to follow up with a neurologist the next day. If he hadn't had a seizure on the way home and returned to the ED, I wonder what would have happened to him.

I took one look at the 12-lead EKG and was concerned. It was alarming to see AV dissociation with a right bundle branch block on a 21-year-old man who had no previous cardiac history. He had no drug abuse history or seizure disorder. Upon questioning, he claimed to have had a fever of 103-104 F 2 weeks prior, accompanied by a rash on his abdomen and back. He was treated with the antibiotic Cipro.

He continued to have seizures while I took over his care. I witnessed his eyes roll back to the right and his arms and legs become rigid. Following these seizures, he had amnesia accompanied by vomiting. I asked the doctor to transfer him to the critical-care area. ICU could accept the patient only if I took care of him because the unit was short-staffed. He then was diagnosed with possible meningitis. I searched high and low for an appropriate cardiac monitor. I gave up and took one from the ICU that would give me an oxygenation saturation reading and a battery for transport. The patient continued to have seizures. By now, they had become more and more frequent, occurring about every 5 minutes and lasting for 5 seconds at a time. I watched him like a hawk.

I asked the ICU monitor technician to record the rhythm just before a seizure. I expected to see a slow heart rate, but I was shocked to see asystole—a straight line! The cardiologist was summoned, and a temporary pacemaker was inserted immediately. He was pacing 100% and totally dependent on the pacemaker. His seizures then terminated. He rested and slept for the rest of the day. I could not stop thinking about him long after I left the ICU that day.

That patient taught me valuable lessons about how to listen and learn. I learned to pay attention to my intuition. I learned that Lyme disease, the patient's diagnosis, must be taken very seriously, as it can cause heart inflammation and serious heart blocks. I learned that in my heart, I will always be a critical-care nurse. I enjoy having the luxury of support staff, time, and proper equipment to help the patient and to be able to appreciate the immediate patient outcome.

PROVIDING CARE ONCE REMOVED
by Allethaire Cullen (Rhode Island, USA)

Usually, I'm sound asleep by 10 p.m., or by 11:01 p.m. if I've been watching *Law and Order* or *ER*. On Thursday, Feb. 20, 2003, I had stayed up to watch *ER*—yet here it was, after midnight, and I was still wide awake. There was no reason for this sleeplessness. I had turned off the television, so I couldn't even claim overstimulation from the news. "This is ridiculous," I muttered to Molly, one of my two cats. Molly was unimpressed. "I'm going to take a shower. Maybe that will relax me."

I would never find out.

When I got out of the shower, Molly was dancing back and forth in front of the bathroom door. Molly—being a nervous cat—is often dancing around about something, but this was different. She was upset. And then I heard it: My pager went off, apparently for the second time.

The caller was my director. "There's a Code 99," she told me, using our phrase for a disaster. "The hospital is expecting 40 victims." She didn't know any more than that.

A disaster with 40 victims should be newsworthy, I thought, so I turned on the television as I dressed. The Station, a local nightclub only miles from the hospital, had been on fire for more than an hour.

As I drove through deserted streets, curiously not stopping once for red light, I listened to reports on the radio. This was big and really, really bad. The Station had been packed with patrons, and the fire, they said, had been intense. Within 3 minutes, the entire building had been engulfed by flames. "Eyewitnesses say there may be several fatalities," a reporter announced in what would later become one of the understatements of the decade. "At the moment, there are no confirmed deaths, but there are many, many injuries."

Governor Don Carcieri likes to say that while most of the world is connected by 6 degrees of separation, in Rhode Island it's more like degree. There was no question that those "many, many injuries" would involve people I knew or knew of. In Rhode Island, we might not all be related—not even cousins once removed—but we're a pretty tightly knit community just the same.

I am an emergency nurse. That's technically not true, because I haven't worked in the emergency department (ED) during the last decade. My skills are rusty, and my protocols are old, and I probably don't even know how to use the new IV tubing. I thought I would be as useful as a flat tire, but in my head, heart, and hands, I'm still an emergency nurse.

That night, however, I wasn't; I was assigned to be a runner attached to public relations (PR). That night, I would not provide care for anyone involved in the disaster. And that, to me, was as unnatural as snow falling up.

I met another member of my department in the hospital parking lot and together we headed down the main concourse. It was eerily empty until we saw a couple of firefighters coming toward us. I remember two things: They were very, very young, and they were smiling. At the time, I thought, "Maybe it isn't as bad as we feared." Later, I realized that they were both in shock.

We made our way to the PR department to get our orders, only to learn that our "runner" jobs already had been completed by people who had been called in earlier. Family members and friends of victims had been herded into the cafeteria next door to the PR office, and they seemed to be the biggest concern at the moment. "Do me a favor," one of the PR people said. "That woman over there, Mrs. Davidson, wants to know what's going on with her son, Thomas. Can you run down to the ED and find out?"

On the way through the ED waiting room and treatment area, I saw many victims walking or sitting up alert, looking relatively unscathed. I noticed the noise but not the smell. Later, I found out that I was probably the only person who didn't. But I did notice a haze in the air, visible and gray, as if every victim had brought in smoke, like a little black cloud. Everything else faded into the background. All I could see were victims with haze.

Thomas was in the medical care unit (MCU), which normally is reserved for 15 acutely ill patients. There were not 15 patients in MCU, but nearly 30 instead. Thomas was in the space reserved for the most acutely ill. He was alert; he was not intubated but had a nonrebreather mask. His face was swathed in gauze and Kerlix, and a surgeon was with him, along with three nurses. Thomas was sitting up, because there was blood pouring from a major laceration on his back. To escape The Station, Thomas had thrown himself through a window, but he had been unable to escape the shards of glass still in the window frame.

I asked the RN in charge of MCU what I could tell Thomas' mother. Almost automatically, she replied, "Tell her he's being evaluated, and it will be some time before she can see him." I had the sense that the poor soul had had to say that 800 times already. I respected her for being able to make it 801.

"Let's try this," I suggested. "The surgeon is with him. He's breathing on his own at the moment, which is a good sign. He has some burns on his face, but he's awake and has been medicated for pain." I also would tell her that it would be several hours before she could see him.

The MCU nurse shrugged and added, "That's probably all his mother could tolerate right now."

"You mean inhalation injury?" I asked.

She nodded. "So far he's breathing on his own, but you know that's not going to last. I don't want to think about what's in these people's lungs."

Neither did I. On my way back to the cafeteria, I rehearsed what I would tell Thomas' mother. "He's breathing on his own so far, but that may change" and "I couldn't see the burns on his face because they were bandaged." But surprisingly, Mrs. Davidson didn't let me say more.

"I don't care," she whispered. "I don't care. I don't care. He's alive." Her eyes lit up. "He's really, truly, alive?"

To this day, I can still hear the hope in her voice, and I can remember how it felt to confirm that hope. It would be the last time I would hear hope for many, many days; it would be the only time I could confirm hope, too.

By about 3 a.m., all the families had either been moved to the ED waiting room or had been sent to Crowne Plaza, a local hotel now serving as command central. My services as a family runner no longer were required.

But PR had a more pressing issue—phone calls. Dozens … hundreds … phone calls from desperate families and friends looking for loved ones. One of the PR staff, a former nursing supervisor, handed me a list of the names of our patients and promised to get lists from other nearby hospitals. "Take a phone," she said. "Do what you can. Don't think of it as answering the phone. Think of it as providing care from a distance." Only a nurse would look at it that way.

The phone that currently was unstaffed was in the PR director's office. The director himself was in and out. There was a small television on a bookshelf, tuned to a local station that had a live picture feed from the scene. The news anchor said, "We do have confirmation of at least one fatality." One, I thought. That cataclysmic inferno and only one victim. The phone rang. Think of it, I reminded myself, as providing care from a distance. Caring, once removed.

"Do you have any information about the victims of the West Warwick fire?" asked a trembling young voice.

"Yes, I do. What's the name of the person you're looking for?"

"My sister, Karen DeLuca."

"Let me check our list." Check it once, check it twice. Do anything not to say "no." But eventually, tell the truth. "No, I'm sorry. Karen DeLuca hasn't been in our emergency department."

There was silence. Then, the young voice pleaded: "What should I do? Please tell me, what should I do?" The last word faded off in a soft wail of despair. What answer is there?

"Have you checked the other hospitals?" I asked, grabbing at anything to keep hope alive. "Let me give you their phone numbers ..."

That scenario would be repeated hundreds of times over the next several hours. We would eventually be able to tell callers, "I have lists from other hospitals, too, so if you find out nothing here, we can try to find your loved one at another ED." Calls came so swiftly that you couldn't let go of the phone when you hung up—before you could remove your hand, the phone would be ringing again. Again and again, the question would come: "What should I do?"

I had a yellow legal pad in front of me. When someone gave me the name of a loved one, I wrote it down before I started searching the lists. I have a memory like a sieve, you see, and I wanted to be sure I made no errors. After a few hours, the paper was covered with names, and I was getting repeat calls from people who were searching for names I'd already failed to find.

That should have triggered something in my mind. I should have realized that if these people were alive, they would have communicated with their loved ones by then. But I didn't realize it, because the local television station had a confirmed report of only one fatality. "Look at all these names," I thought to myself. "They can't all be fatalities. So far there's only one." Please, God, these were just kids who missed curfew, who had escaped the fire but were still stunned, who had gone to a different club ... anything but what, in retrospect, seems so obvious. Anything but that they were dead. After all, there was only one reported fatality.

One became 26. The reporters updated their stories as dawn approached. One of the network's early morning shows had sent a mobile truck to do a story in front of our hospital. The local news stations all had reporters outside. Early-to-bed people were just waking up to the news, and the phones started ringing with new vigor. People who hadn't realized their loved ones might be in danger woke up to fear. By that point, though, the phone calls were asking for the same names over and over. I didn't have to keep going through the lists, even though I did. I knew. Twenty-six dead. I had far more than 26 names on my pad, and the grisly reality began to sink in: Many of them, maybe most of them, were dead, or else they would have contacted their loved ones.

It was then that I realized I was not just passing on information; it was far worse than that. I was taking away hope. These callers would try to contact their loved ones first. They would call around everywhere before they would call us. But eventually, they would call us. "No, I'm sorry; I can't find his name on any of the hospitals' lists." I wanted to add, "But don't give up hope! Maybe he's still at the site, watching the fire. Maybe she's at a friend's house. Maybe …" But I said none of those things, because they would have been lies. I could not give false hope. I could only take hope away.

Think of it as caring from a distance. If this phone call was the first step on the road of grief, it became my responsibility to make it one of edification—to make sure that this phone call was somehow a positive thing. That sounds so bizarre, but any nurse will understand. When we have to break bad news to a patient's family, we try to do so in a positive, supportive, and compassionate manner. The family becomes our patient. We nurse the loved ones. And even though I was geographically removed from these people, my role was the same. My role was to care, even at a distance; to care, not close up, but one step removed.

It was very, very difficult. I kept thinking with envy of my former colleagues, the emergency nurses. They had patients in front of them. A touch, some repositioning, gentle words, a well-timed intervention—they could see the fruits of their labors or, at the very least, know that their efforts were the most that could be done. Over and over, I was left with the fact that there were thousands of hurting, grieving, devastated people all over the state, and I was doing nothing for any of them. Perhaps it was the height of arrogance that made me think I could have done something for them, but that's what I believed. I tried to convey the compassion and concern they needed, but their pain was raw and untouched by my efforts. I wanted, as Paul McCartney sang, to "take a sad song and make it better." But the truth was, this song was going to be sad, and nothing would make it better.

Around 9:30 a.m., someone came to relieve me. I tore off the page where I'd written so many names and slipped it into my pocket. Then I went downstairs to pick up my coat. Oddly, I was reluctant to go home. I puttered around a deserted office for a while. It was as if I couldn't tear myself away. The worst was over for us, but I didn't want to leave.

I walked into my house around 10:30 a.m., greeted by two cranky, hungry cats Breakfast was more than 5 hours late, and nothing, not even a devastating fire, took precedence over breakfast as far as they were concerned. Automatically, I took off my coat and fed them. The smell of raw fish in the Fancy Feast actually helped clear my sleep-deprived head.

I called a friend, Lynn, who had worked the ED. It was then that I saw the news flash across the TV screen: 40 confirmed dead, with more anticipated. Lynn heard my gasp. She had spoken with several fire-fighters that night, so it was no surprise to her. "Allie, they think there might be a hundred dead."

I thought of the names on my list, now tucked inside my purse. When it was one fatality, I thought those people might be alive. Now, I knew that virtually none of them was.

All through the day and night, the local stations continued coverage of the fire. The number of dead crept up: 67, 82, 97. On Saturday, as medical examiners identified the bodies, officials started releasing names of those who had perished. Within a week, all the names had been released. I began to highlight names on my list, names of the dead. Soon, it became difficult to find a name that was not highlighted.

During those days, I began to redefine my list. In the beginning, it was a list of failure. It was a list of all those families and friends who I had been unable to help. I'm a nurse! I'm supposed to make things better! This was a list representing those for whom I'd had to steal hope. I had tried to provide care, even if it had been from a distance. But what good was that? These people were dead. The people who called me were bereft.

But as the days passed, I came to view my list differently. Yes, it was a collection of the names of victims, but it was so much more than that. All the people on that list, I began to see, had had people who loved them. I know that, because I spoke to the people who loved them, who tried to find them at 3 a.m., who begged to know what else they could do to find them. Maybe from my selfish perspective, the list was one of personal failure. But in reality, it was a list of profound, lasting, and unwavering love—of transcendent love. And really, between failure and love, which one of those two should endure?

Sixteen days after the fire, I brought that list and some flowers to the site of The Station fire. Hundreds of others had been there before me.

The chain link fence surrounding the site was covered with flowers, teddy bears, photos, T-shirts, and other forms of remembrance honoring the dead. I placed my flowers and the list at a spot near a photo collage of a girl whose name I recognized—a name from my list, a highlighted name.

It seemed only right to decorate a place where so much pain, fear, horror, and loss abounded. Shouldn't there be some reminders that in the midst of all that, there was love? That's what the teddy bears and other mementos meant to those who left them; that's what my list meant to me. And if I couldn't care for the victims directly, I could at least express my caring through their friends' and families' love. It was caring that was not given directly, but was once removed.

Caring once removed is often the way nurses care for their patients. This kind of caring goes on for days, for months, for years later. It is what nurses live and believe, but really don't talk about. It hurts too much. So much of nursing hurts too much. Nurses know how to help those who need this special work. But who helps the nurse with grief? Is it just a given that he or she will get over it? Countless words on the pages of this book show that nurses continue to feel grief and loss deeply. They can't let their patients go.

Nurse researchers have documented that after a child's death, bereaved parents say they must move on, but they don't actually let go completely (Murphy, Johnson, & Lohan, 2003). That child remains in their hearts forever. Nurses who work in critical care will also tell you that when a child dies, they are left speechless. It is a time of struggle— a time of guilt, blame, and anger. The flood of emotions the family must deal with is unrivaled. The mental distress, depression, and grief that follow are agonizing. The reality of the loss is consuming. It is the same for the nurse.

INITIATING HEROIC ACTIONS
by Jana Bartkova (Kezmarok, Slovakia)

I would like to introduce to you what I consider to be the heroic actions of nurses in Slovakia, who with hard work and enthusiasm have opened the first agencies of home healthcare in Slovakia. Since the change of the political systems after 1989 and the ensuing transformation of healthcare and the example of Western countries, we have started opening home healthcare agencies.

There were many problems in the beginning. Doctors and health insurance companies did not understand the purpose of the project. Health insurance companies were not able to understand that care for patients in their homes is much cheaper than expensive hospitalization. We encountered these barriers in the hospital of Kezmarok, a city located beneath the Tatra's mountains. We were able to cross these barriers only because we believed that we were doing this for the people who need this care the most, our patients.

We understood that our home healthcare was not only economically better but also very humane for our patients. We understood that the home environment gives our patients a feeling of security, comfort, faith, and hope. I confess that there were moments when we wanted to give up. It was only the thought of our patients who needed our services, that gave us the enthusiasm and strength to continue.

We still have not yet crossed all the barriers. After 2 years in our agency, though, we do see that we are really fulfilling our patient's needs. This shows in the many thankful letters that we have received from our patients and their families. This is the highest moral prize for our week.

I would like to also say that not every nurse is able to work for a home healthcare agency. A nurse who works for a home healthcare agency should be professional and have high morals. I am very happy to say in Kezmarok we have many nurses with such high standards. It is because of such nurses from this little but beautiful country in the heart of Europe that I am able to write such a story. In the same way that Florence Nightingale brought with her lamp of hope for the suffering, nurses from our agency are bringing the light of hope to the homes of our patients.

From the bottom of my heart, I wish to all the patients in the whole world that they will receive care from exceptional nurses like Florence Nightingale, nurses like those in our agency in Kezmarok. In our hard work we always go by the motto: By taking care of the happiness of other people we are finding our own.

INITIATING A GIFT OF LIFE FOR OTHERS
by Sharon Saunderson Cohen (Florida, USA)

My pager announced that another trauma would soon be arriving at the trauma resuscitation unit. With each alert, I think of all the preparation that nurses, physicians, and staff go through to be ready for any and every patient who may need care. I responded as usual, with a bit of trepidation and a lot of adrenaline. This particular case gave me a sour-gut feeling. As I have matured as a nurse, I have learned to trust my gut. It rarely proves me wrong.

Arriving at the trauma resuscitation unit was a 12-year-old girl who, only minutes before, had been waiting for the school bus to take her home after a full day at school. Now, in the hectic and often insane pace of the trauma resuscitation unit, a petite girl restrained on a backboard, with IVs in both arms and a breathing tube, arrived with a most peaceful look upon her face. I remember thinking that Tina looked far too peaceful to be so critically injured. Her face didn't have a scratch. In fact, she had only small lacerations on her arm and leg. She looked so angelic amidst the intensity of the environment.

The initial assessment indicated that Tina was in an extremely critical state. Her pupils were unequal, with one being fixed and the other sluggishly trying to react to my penlight. She did not have any respiratory effort other than what was provided by the ventilator, and her blood pressure was too low to provide for adequate blood flow to her brain. Our actions had to be swift, for each second counted and each intervention was with life-saving intent.

Based on the quick assessment, IV fluids were changed to include medications to help the brain function better, and an emergent trip for a CT scan was underway. The whole trauma team was desperately trying to save this little girl's life. It amazes me that five to eight people can descend upon a critically injured patient, work together like a well-oiled machine, and produce amazing results. Tina needed every part of this machine working on her behalf to keep her alive. For a brief moment, I wondered if anyone had found the child's mother to let her know the seriousness of her daughter's injuries. My heart began to sink as Tina, our little angelic-looking but severely injured patient, rapidly began to take a turn for the worse. Her vital signs were worsening, and despite every effort to stabilize her condition, her brain was beginning to shut down. Again I wondered about Tina's mom. I made a quick call to the trauma resuscitation unit, but they couldn't locate the mother. The police, I was told, were unable to locate her before emergency medical services transported Tina to the hospital.

At some point in my nursing career, I began to understand and accept that not all trauma patients can be saved. In my earlier years as a nurse, I felt that if I worked hard enough, if I worked smart enough, then any patient could be saved. I often harbored anger if a patient died—anger aimed at myself. I thought I wasn't a good nurse. I thought that I should be smarter, that I should work more efficiently—I should be one step ahead of the patient's clinical course. If I did all this, then patients would not and could not die. I tormented myself for many years before a co-worker and mentor helped me see that sometimes my efforts weren't in vain, even if the patient died. She helped me see that many of my efforts could be directed to the families and loved ones who had to come to terms with the loss of someone who meant so much to them.

The CT scan confirmed our worst fears. Tina had suffered an inoperable and severe brain injury that we were almost certain she couldn't survive. I was desperate to find Tina's mother. I didn't know how long we could keep Tina alive, despite the efforts of so many. From the trauma resuscitation unit, we took her to the pediatric intensive care unit (PICU), where the feverish pace of trying to keep the small girl alive continued. Knowing that I was transferring Tina into very competent nursing hands, I turned my energies to locating her mother. After many inquiries, I got a call from the local police department. Tina's mother, Sheila, had been located. She was working in a city 30 minutes away and was being brought to the hospital.

Despite continued assessments and interventions in the PICU, the brain flow study told us that Tina's brain had not been able to handle the impact of the injury. She was brain dead. The atmosphere in Tina's room was solemn, but work continued at a constant pace. As nurses, we all felt the same emotions. We had all tried, with every bit of knowledge and every ounce of energy, to save her life. I addressed the topic of organ donation with the staff. Even if our efforts to save Tina were futile, we still could hope that the gift of life could be given to others if Sheila would consent to organ donation.

Finally, Sheila arrived. We took her to a quiet room so she could have some privacy as we explained her daughter's situation. As I walked to the room where Sheila was sitting, I could see how much Tina resembled her mother. Oh how I wished she could understand that Tina was okay now. All the pain and hard work were over. Though Tina was brain dead, I knew in my gut she had reached a higher place that allowed her peace. When I told her, "Your child has died," I, too, nearly died as I saw the forlorn look on her face turn to deep pain and anguish. We all felt it. It's a pain unlike any other—the kind that pierces the heart.

Thank God for another gut feeling. Sometimes I truly feel that my days are dictated by my gut. I really believed that Sheila needed to see her daughter, not listen to how hard we tried to save her or how severe her head injury was. The great nurses at organ procurement supported me as I walked Sheila to her daughter's room. The PICU nurses were ready for Sheila and greeted her with gentle smiles and warm touches. Sheila talked to her as she stroked her daughter's hair and face. We left them alone to absorb the moment. Slowly, we noticed the look of pain fade from Sheila's face. After several moments, she turned and asked: "How do I make sense of this? My baby is gone."

I took her shaking hand in mine. As tears rolled down her cheeks and mine, I introduced the idea of organ donation. Though Tina's brain could not keep her alive, her heart was still beating, and the rest of her organs were uninjured. We talked for several minutes about options in organ donation and about how the tragedy of Tina's death could offer the gift of life for others. Amazingly, Sheila told us about a conversation she had had about a year before with her precious, insightful daughter.

After school one day, Tina had told her mother about a visitor to her classroom who had spoken to them about his experience: He was alive because someone had died and that person's family had donated the deceased's organs. Tina was amazed at this guest's courage, and she said if something should ever happen to her, she wanted to give somebody her heart. Sheila said she hadn't taken Tina's wish seriously, until that day.

Slowly, I could see Sheila's aching easing somewhat as she agreed to allow her daughter's wish to come true. Tina, as insightful as she was, gave her heart and other organs to six other people. Though her daughter was gone, the gift of life and the miracle of making a little girl's wish come true helped Sheila find some sense of meaning in her precious daughter's death.

Although the trauma team and I couldn't change the final outcome, I truly feel we found meaning in Tina's death and helped her mother do so as well. While trying to save the little girl's life, all of our clinical decisions were correct. We acted efficiently and were one step ahead of Tina's clinical course, until her brain couldn't overcome the injury anymore. We tried, but we didn't fail. What we did was allow Sheila to feel that something good came from something so devastating. Our interventions didn't help keep Tina alive, but they did help her mother begin the healing process.

In nursing, I have been taught about the grieving process. I do not practice nursing in a vacuum, nor do I begin to heal in a vacuum. It takes the whole trauma team to keep a victim alive. It takes the whole team to help a parent cope with the loss of a child. It takes the whole team to help each other through the process of death. It took the whole team to assist this young mother in grieving over the loss of her only daughter, and through that, to help save the lives of six people.

DOING WHAT HAD NOT BEEN DONE BEFORE
by Monica Dancu (Florida, USA)

We received a 21-year-old female patient from the intensive care unit (ICU) following a car accident. She had been delivering newspapers to make extra money for the family. Her husband usually watched their 2-year-old daughter, but that morning he had a job interview. So, the woman put her daughter in the car seat, and off to work they went. Not long after, an accident occurred. The mother sustained multiple injuries, including a right acetabular fracture, and her daughter was killed. Her husband took the loss very hard and blamed himself for the daughter's death. The ICU nurses convinced him to spend the night at the hospital.

When the mother was moved to the Step Down unit, she told the nurses she would love to see her baby one more time. The nurses talked to her husband, her parents, the hospital chaplain, and the funeral director. All felt that attending a funeral service would be important in helping the mother achieve closure. I don't know if this had ever been done before, but we held a funeral service in her room. Family members and friends arrived at the hospital. The staff took them to a waiting area at the end of the hall. Shortly thereafter, the funeral director and hospital chaplain arrived, carrying a small white casket with gold handles and angels. The beautiful little girl had not a mark on her, and she looked as if she were sleeping. Her grandma put a Precious Moments angel necklace on her. Because the little girl loved butterflies, pink ones were placed inside the casket, and her aunt put gold butterflies on the outside.

The funeral director put the casket next to the mother's bed. Her cervical collar and pulse oximeter were removed, so she could turn her head to see the baby and hold her daughter's hand one last time. Everyone started to cry when the mother said her daughter's hand was so cold.

The nurses left the room, and the service started. When it was over, everyone except the parents left the room. The family thanked me for the help and encouragement I provided. The nurses truly made a difference by making sure the patient got her wish. I'm so proud of all of these nurses who made this experience possible for a mother who had such a tremendous loss.

PROVIDING CARE THAT CHANGED A LIFE
by Gloria H. Denston (Florida, USA)

Fifteen years ago, a teenager named Steve was admitted with severe compound fractures of his right lower extremity from a motorcycle accident. The injuries were severe, and his physician and our nurses were gravely concerned that he might lose his leg. While we planned how to restore function to his leg and clear the infection, Steve concerned himself with getting out and restoring his motorcycle so he could ride again.

At first, he was impatient with his healing and the need for repeated surgeries. Like most teenagers, he believed himself invincible, and he was full of denial. He refused to look at his leg wounds and wanted the leg covered at all times. His youthful optimism, however, eventually gave way to concerns about his slow healing.

Providing care for Steve while he was optimistic was easy, as he would joke and tease with us for his entertainment. He did not know

of our deep concerns for his leg. As the weeks passed with more sur
geries for Steve, his needs changed. He feared the pain of dressing
changes and repeated surgeries. His fear caused him at times to act ou
and refuse dressing changes. I became one of his principal caregiver
for consistency of care. I became the nurse, surrogate mother, and
friend, finding it difficult at times to keep the role of nurse first.

With dressing changes, I would pre-medicate him to lessen the pain
As the repeated surgeries were scheduled, I would listen to his con
cerns and fears. When reality set in that he might lose his leg, I held his
hand while the physician explained the gravity of his situation. And
when Steve just wanted to cry, I found myself crying with him. He
talked about his dreams and the things he would not be able to do.
found myself encouraging him to look at how lucky he was to still have
his leg, and reminded him of all he could do. When boredom set in afte
weeks in his room, we moved his bed into the hall by the nurse's sta
tion, so he could socialize. We decorated his overhead frame and trac
tion with balloons and signs that said, "Tickle my foot." He found that
particularly funny.

Steven was very lucky, and after long weeks of skilled care, surgeries
and physical therapy, he was well enough to go home and continue
with his wound care. The leg was weak, and he needed 6 months o
rehabilitation.

When Steven left the hospital, it was like I had lost a child. I worried
how he would make out with his rehab. I wondered if he would
remember my words of encouragement and continue to see the cup as
half full instead of half empty. More importantly, I worried that he
would let this injury be an excuse not to live a full life.

Initially, Steven kept in touch with me, visiting whenever he had fol
low-up visits with his physician. Years passed with fewer and fewer vis
its. I wondered how my Steven would adjust as an adult.

This past year, Steven came to see me in the post anesthesia care unit (PACU). You cannot imagine my surprise, as this young teenager had grown into a 6-foot-tall man. He was now married with a daughter of his own. But the biggest surprise was that he was wearing a sheriff's officer uniform. I wondered how he had been able to endure the physical training required. Steven told me how he had worked out with the goal of making it on the police force. He had been determined not to let his injuries stop him from realizing his dreams. My eyes welled with tears and my heart filled with pride as I remembered saying those very same words to him many years earlier.

A person never knows how an encounter or experience may influence a life, but I do know Steven and I must have connected, since he came back to show me what he had accomplished. When Steven lifted his uniform pants to show me how his injured leg had healed, the scars were not ugly to me, but rather a wonderful testament to a young boy's determination and the skill of nursing care provided by numerous healthcare providers years earlier. Steven told me he has never forgotten his care and the crazy stunts we did to him. My nursing career has given me such wonderful satisfaction—being able to see the benefits of my work and that of my colleagues in nursing.

HELPING A SON MAKE CONTACT
by Irene Quiles (New Jersey, USA)

The man walked into our unit each afternoon as the winter sun was setting. He always looked the same—he wore a hooded sweatshirt, a flannel shirt, jeans, and work boots splattered with cement. He entered his mother's room, carrying a newspaper. He would greet her, sit down, and silently read the paper. She knew he was there, yet she never acknowledged him. After an hour, he would say goodbye and leave. This woman did not lack the ability to communicate, nor did she lack the cognition to know who he was; she always spoke with staff as they cared for her.

The disease that was robbing her of her life advanced quickly. On her last day, the construction worker arrived as always. He did not read his paper. He called for the nurse. He asked but one thing of me, and I was unsure if I could do what he asked and not betray my patient. He wanted to hold her, one last time. The tears welled in his eyes, and his voice shook. Perhaps this would heal whatever rift kept her silent when her only visitor came each day. Her breathing was shallow and irregular. There was no time for an ethical discussion.

In my heart, I knew there was no choice. The son was already removing the blankets from his mother. Together we untangled oxygen, IV lines, and bed coverings. He sat on the bed, and we moved her into his arms. He cradled her gently, kissing her forehead and crying. A flash of Michelangelo's "Pietà" came to me. Time stopped in the room. She looked into his face and smiled—the smile a mother gives a child when together they overcome an obstacle that was a Herculean task. Was it a minute? An hour? I cannot tell you what segment of time passed, but when her soul left her body, the mother granted peace to her son. Together we placed her on the bed, and he covered her and stroked her hair. He left as he always did—newspaper under his arm, walking into the winter darkness.

Nurses in the operating room (OR) are a specialty group with incredible knowledge. Their ability to prepare for and assist in the surgical setting is wide-ranging. Always on call and adaptable to swift change, these nurses provide expert care. The patients may never know these nurses; they often are foggy remembrances. For some, however, the nurse-patient connection is striking, and long-lasting friendships are built.

Knowledge of instruments, high tech machinery, oxygenation indicators, and pharmacological agents, as well as strict sterile technique, is innate to OR nurses. It is team nursing, requiring complete connection with the surgical team: scrub nurse, heart/lung technician, circulating nurse, first assistant, and surgeon. The synchrony of the work is exquisite, each nurse instrumental in assisting with a surgical masterpiece.

REMOVING THE FEAR
by Nancy Boyd (Florida, USA)

My patient was a 14-year-old girl. Debby was very petite, but she seemed so muscular at first appearance. Later, I learned the reason why. I wondered why she was having back surgery. Why was she having an anterior lumbar interbody fusion? This is a major abdominal operation to restore a spine damaged by degenerative disc disease. It is one thing to know you will be assisting in surgery on an older person begging for relief from intractable pain, or a trauma patient with a fractured spine who may be partially paralyzed. But to see a child having this procedure made me uncomfortable. So, I looked at the x-rays and soon discovered the reason. She had the back of a 60-year-old woman. Immediately, I refocused myself and began the process I love so much—being a patient advocate.

First, I introduced myself as the specialty coordinator for spines. I told her I would be her nurse in surgery—that I would be with her the whole time. I was recalling Maslow's hierarchy of needs from nursing school and psychology. Safety and security were crucial in the thought processes. I asked her name and birth date, while looking at her armband to verify the information imprinted. She responded, ever so softly, "Debby."

I said, "I had a best friend named Debby, so we'll get along famously." She smiled and started to laugh, just a little. I told her that I would be asking her a lot of questions that would be necessary for her care, and she just rolled her eyes. After we finished the usual medical history, began to tell her about the procedure. At this point, she started to cry. I grabbed her hand and held it tight, like a mother would do, and then told her I had three boys and one girl. She asked my daughter's name and I said, "Angela." She replied, "Oh goody." That was her best friend's name, so again we had something in common. She blurted out the same remark I had said. "We'll get along famously." I laughed. She seemed to relax a bit. I told her that she would go back to the operating room on the stretcher. It would be very cold, but we would place special warm blankets over her. She then questioned if I would keep her covered up as she was so modest. I remembered how my daughter was at 14, just showing signs of maturity, so I told her that I would protect her as if she were my own daughter. At this time, her mother and father just looked at me. I smiled at them and acknowledged their concerns.

She told me she was a gymnast, and I realized that this accounted for her muscular build. Debby said she wanted very much to compete, and her goal was to be on the United States Olympic team. I listened. My body became tense, knowing what would come next. She then grabbed my hand and asked, "Can I compete after surgery?" I asked Debby what her doctor had told her, and she quickly said in a monotone voice, as if she had memorized lines from a play: "We have to take one day at a time. You are young and healthy. Everything is possible."

Debby then looked deep in my eyes and asked, "Is that true?"

"Indeed it is true that you will have to take one day at a time, and you will get stronger and more confident as the days pass," I said. "You are definitely young and healthy. Keep in mind that it will not be easy, but for a competitor like you, it will be your newest hurdle to jump." All this time she was nodding as if in agreement.

Then she asked me what kind of scars she would have on her belly. Could she wear her new bikini? I told her that if everything proceeded the way we expected and there were no unexpected occurrences, she could wear her bikini. Her mom then joined in and said, "See, I told you so." So again, there was a chuckle from all except the father.

Debby then asked if I had ever been on a team that performed this type of surgery on someone her age. I responded that I had not, but that I had assisted with the operation on several 16- and 17-year-old athletes who had gone on to do very well. She enthusiastically said, "Well, okay, then I'm yours." I breathed a huge sigh of relief. Recalling nursing theory, I had told her the truth and used my experiences to gain her confidence.

At this point, her father, who had sat silently in the corner, peered up from his reading glasses while clutching a medical journal and asked in a quivering voice, "Nancy, if you had to have this type of surgery, would you trust the surgeon and staff?" Again, I was taken by surprise. I then walked around the stretcher, grasped his hand firmly, and said, "Most definitely."

He then said, "Well, you can take my little girl now." By this time, Dad, Mom, Debby, and I all had tears in our eyes. After this, I unlocked the stretcher, and we were off on our journey. Now, take into consideration that all of this took place in our pre-surgery area in a time span of approximately 15 minutes, which can seem like a lifetime for the nurses and family. Can you imagine the uncertainty that faced this family and their willingness to surrender their lives to us? This demonstrates

the immense role of the nurse in the operating room. We are patien
advocates. We are totally responsible for their nursing care—what
truly awesome role.

Debby entered the surgical suite and had her operation under th
expert care of two surgeons, an anesthesiologist, and operating roon
personnel. She had textbook results. With the surgical procedure com
pleted, relief filled the once-silent room. Immediately afterward, witl
permission from the surgeons, I went to speak to the family in the sur
gical waiting room. I told them that Debby had done extremely well
but that it would be one day at a time.

MAKING THE EFFORT TO SET PRIORITIES
by Rebecca Hilgen Bryan (New Jersey, USA)

I was assigned that day to Jonah, a family man who was dying from
failed liver transplant. I was working in the surgical intensive care uni
(ICU), where we prided ourselves on taking care of the sickest peopl
in the city. This man was teetering on the edge of his life. That day wa
a big day, I was told in report. We were to make him look as well as pos
sible, because his children were coming in to say goodbye.

Because of high ammonia levels and medications, Jonah was waftin
in and out of sleep. He was quite yellow, and his drain had leaked a lit
tle on his gown, though of course the night shift had left him with
spotless bed and body. I thought the best thing to do was to hide a
much of the technical equipment as I could, to avoid scaring the chil
dren. They were due in at 10 a.m. I wrote my assessment, adjuste
Jonah's meds, changed his gown, and straightened his room.

It was 9:30 a.m. when the surgical resident trudged in, looking as if he had been up all night. "Prep him for a spinal tap to check for infection." As usual, there was no "hello" or "how are you doing?" I told him the spinal tap would have to wait, as the family was due in half an hour and this was a big day. He gave me a derogatory look and said it had to happen now! He had no time the rest of the day. It wouldn't take long, and then he'd be out of my hair. I thought of the mess, the bed to remake, and the instruments to quickly dispose of so as not to scare the children, but I kept my mouth closed as I went to get the surgical kit. I held Jonah's sagging, frail body against mine as we propped him up on the side of the bed. I spoke comforting words as the resident inserted the needle into his back. Then I watched as his blood pressure first shot up, then went down, along with his oxygen saturation. The needle had missed its target, puncturing his lung. Since coagulopathy was among his terminal ailments, Jonah began to bleed and suffocate. A code was called. About the same time, the unit secretary informed me that his family had arrived and was out in the hall.

Others ran the code; I was the connection with the family. Jonah's young daughters were dressed in their Sunday best. I pulled his wife aside and told her there had been a complication. They remained hopeful and patiently waited down the hall. I went back to the unit—the code was a mess. They were using the defibrillator. They were pushing every medication in the book. The transplant surgeon, a kind man with large black eyes, kept encouraging the code team. The bed—heck, the whole room—was a huge mess. It was obvious that Jonah was dead. This time I was crying as I spoke with his wife. She still had some hope. I went back into the unit, walked up to the transplant surgeon, and said: "He's gone. How long can they code him? You have to speak to the family." He looked at me, looked at Jonah, and then called the code. He walked heavily out to the waiting room. The surgical resident couldn't look me in the eye.

My coworkers helped as I made Jonah and his room look as presentable as possible. We did a pretty good job, only now he was dead. Two hours after they were expecting to see their loved one, the family said goodbye to Jonah. It was heart-wrenching, as I felt torn between grief for the family and anger at the resident.

That surgical resident actually came up later that afternoon and apologized to me. That surprised me—I didn't think he had it in him. Of course, I wasn't the one who was owed the apology: Jonah and his family were. I told him that. And I told him about priorities. You know what? It's been at least 12 years since that happened. And I hold that to this day as my standard for keeping priorities straight.

RESPONDING TO A SENSE OF UNEASINESS
by Jean Werner (Florida, USA)

Mr. T was 45 years old—handsome, robust, and youthful-looking. He told me that he had been hit by a car while riding his bike across the street. A health-conscious man, he was returning home after a trip to the health food store.

I noticed he had a glassy look in his eyes. Even though he appeared to be stable, I had an all-too-familiar uneasiness come over me that he was much sicker than his appearance. I pulled the curtain and began to assess him. When I pulled down his sheet, I could see pins coming out of his pelvic areas that had been placed to stabilize his fractures. But most troubling was a generalized redness of his entire lower abdomen that extended down his left leg and also into his scrotal area. There was also some edema there.

I talked with his bedside nurse, and we checked all his labs. A general practitioner physician and an orthopedic surgeon were on his case. We called both of them after our discussion about the redness and swelling. They both said they would check him on rounds. Our day was a usual day in progressive care unit (PCU), very demanding and busy. His nurse had talked to both of these physicians when they made their rounds, but they didn't say much about the redness and swelling. As the day progressed, he remained stable, but the redness and swelling increased.

That uneasiness I had felt earlier was still there, and my frustration level began to rise. I knew something was wrong, but because his numbers weren't too bad, we would just watch him. Dr. A., our internist, made rounds later that day—which is usually when they come to our unit, as we are progressive care, not intensive care. The physician believed the patient had a staph infection of some type. I went home that evening feeling uneasy.

The next morning, we were short-staffed. Not only was I in charge, but I also had a full patient load. Mr. T. was my patient. That morning when I went to see him, he had extreme lower abdominal pain. I pulled back his covers and could not believe what I saw. His entire lower abdomen, his upper left thigh, and his scrotum were swollen tight. In fact, his skin was so tight it was starting to flake. I immediately called Dr. A. I told him my findings and said he would have to come to PCU first thing. He moaned and groaned, but he knew me well enough to know I don't panic easily. When he came into the room and examined Mr. T, he immediately ordered a CT of the abdomen and multiple labs, and he told Mr. T that he thought he had necrotizing fasciitis. He immediately consulted a surgeon and an infection control physician. Performing the CT was very difficult, as any movement was painful for him. As soon as we returned, I hung a morphine drip, which helped control his pain. The diagnosis was confirmed by noon. The surgeon explained to Mr. T that he was to be transferred to Tampa General Hospital. The surgery he needed was extensive. They would have to open up his lower abdomen, leg, penis, and scrotum, or the swelling would compromise his tissue. Mr. T was absolutely overwhelmed by this point. After all the doctors left, he asked me to stay. He wanted to know what I thought of all this. He said, "I don't want to be filleted like a fish." I held his hand and told him I trusted the doctors who had seen him, and if it were my husband, I would have him go to Tampa. He thought about it, and the next time I went into the room he said, "Let's do it." Even though he had all these physical issues going on, his next big problem had nothing to do with his health: He had no insurance. Since this was July 4, it might be next to impossible to find a Tampa physician who would accept him into the system. I worked feverishly the next 6 hours. I called social service workers, nursing administrators, and physicians, trying to coordinate the transfer. Luck was on Mr. T's side that day. Dr. J knew a surgeon in Tampa who knew the surgeon on this case. After making more phone calls and talking with the emergency medical services (EMS) supervisor, we made the arrangements. Mr. T would go to Tampa that night.

As the day progressed, Mr. T was getting more and more septic. He began running a temperature, and his swelling was getting worse. So was his pain. Even on the morphine drip, he was uncomfortable. We increased his dosage, which helped somewhat. The only family he had there was a girlfriend. As the day wore on, she was getting more and more fragile—as was he. I knew time was of the essence. It was like putting together a puzzle. Once I finally found all the edge pieces, I could start filling in the middle. And once the designs and colors were together, the pieces all started to fit. The last piece was the phone call I received from the admitting office in Tampa. He would be accepted, and they would take him that night. I left around 9 p.m., and he left shortly thereafter. I was extremely worried that we had waited too long to send him. But being a believer in fate, I put my trust in the universe. The next time I went to work, I heard that Mr. T had an E. coli necrotizing fasciitis from a perforated rectum. They had done extensive surgery, and he was critical.

I continued to keep a check on him through our social service worker. His progress was slow, but sure. After staying in the hospital for more than 3 months, he came home, walking with a cane. I recently learned that he is doing better physically, but that he had to sell his home and lost his job due to physical limitations. He no longer has the girlfriend, and he is living with a friend. I firmly believe that had he not been in extremely good health when this happened to him, he would not have survived. And, I also believe that if he hadn't been transferred that day, his fate might have been the same.

EVERYONE KNOWS A JOHN DOE
by Debbie Tchorz (Florida, USA)

John Doe, was a young man in his 20s who had fallen victim to a drunk driver. He had been riding his bicycle at the time of the accident, and he had sustained a serious head injury that would later prove fatal.

He had no identification. He was your average handsome Joe. His hair was dark brown and framed his face nicely. He could have been my brother, whom I deeply adore. Adventurous, fun loving, and popular, my brother Joe would take a spin on his bike to catch the wind in his face just to get away from the frustrations and negativity of the world.

As the day progressed, John's condition deteriorated. Sustaining him became a difficult task. No family or friends called or came to the hospital. Even with numerous public agencies helping out, we could not locate his next-of-kin. I knew this was someone's son and someone's loved one. I could not imagine dying in such a desolate way, with no one to comfort me, no one caring, no one saying goodbye. As a nurse, a caregiver, and a patient advocate, there is a connection you have to make. I made this connection with John Doe.

Getting more frantic to find his family, and knowing the police were over loaded with work, I asked that the hospital's public relations group request that a description of John Doe be aired on the local television stations in hopes of someone recognizing him. To my amazement, the request was declined. I was told it wasn't my job to find patients' families.

Through the day, my protective instincts grew deeper and deeper. It was my job to help my patients in the ways they needed. John Doe needed to have someone with him.

After much discussion, it was agreed to air John's description along with some—not all—personal distinctions. I was anxious and excited, but I was afraid as well. What if after all this work and hope, no one came forward? I wept as I watched the critically ill young man sleep. I wondered if our positions were reversed would anyone care enough to look for my loved ones. John Doe's situation and the lack of empathy I had encountered in fighting for him left me feeling sad and vulnerable.

After the news aired, phone calls came pouring in, but none provided strong leads. People from all walks of life came to the hospital offering assistance or following up on what they thought was a lead. In all these people, not one person knew John. I left that evening feeling like a failure. Guidance was what I wanted, but it was the truth that I ached for.

The next morning, I thought of having a sketch of John drawn and then airing the sketch. Again, this suggestion was declined. By now, John had been declared brain dead.

I was angry and annoyed, and I kept thinking that there must be a way! I was outraged too. I could not believe the audacity and the unmitigated gall that people in charge could not support every reasonable, feasible attempt to help John's family find him and be with him.

There was finally a lead from an anonymous caller. I called the number, but it was a landscaping company. I hung up not knowing what to do. I had expected a person not a company. With guilt as my persuader, I phoned back. I discovered that John Doe had worked for the company for a brief time. The owner did provide me with the emergency contact numbers John had provided to them for their personnel files. Anxiously, I called his brother but was not able to reach him. My next plan of attack was the phone book. Now that I knew his real name, I could look for his family. The first call to someone with the same last name as John was a dead end—they had never heard of him. The second call was to his mother. I was sweating and my heart raced as I spoke with her and explained the situation. I had finally succeeded; John's family would arrive shortly.

It was at the very end of my shift that John's mother and father arrived. Recognizing my voice, they approached and asked how I had found them. Holding back the tears, I gave them my answer. Later that evening, John's parents agreed to donate his organs which helped more than five individuals.

That night, I went to bed satisfied and fulfilled. I had performed my job and my expectations to the fullest. I felt no guilt about what I had done. I thought about my brother and telephoned him just to say hello. My last thought that night was "this is what my profession is about—caring not only for the dying but for the living as well.

The ED, the ICU, and the OR are just a few of the places you will find critical care nurses performing their craft. They are scientific thinkers with a keen awareness for the sickest of the sick. It is their observational skills that often save lives or make life better for many. It is their love of nurse work that helps them continue. What we take from these stories is the knowledge that these nurses are truly talented professionals with great power, courage, and strength. Their gifts are many—skillful hands, powerful intuition, and gutsy advocacy. Through it all, they are heroes who won't take "no" for an answer. Never.

REFERENCES

Davidhizar, R., & Shearer, R. (2002). Helping children cope with public disaster. AJN, 102(3), 26-33.

Gebbie, K., & Qureshi, K. (2002). Emergency and disaster preparedness. AJN, 102(1), 46-51.

Murphy, S.A., Johnson, L.C., & Lohan, J. (2003). Challenging the myths about parents' adjustment after the sudden, violent death of a child. Journal of Nursing Scholarship, 35(4), 359-364.

Steinhauer, R. (2002). Bioterrorism. RN, 65(3), 48-55.

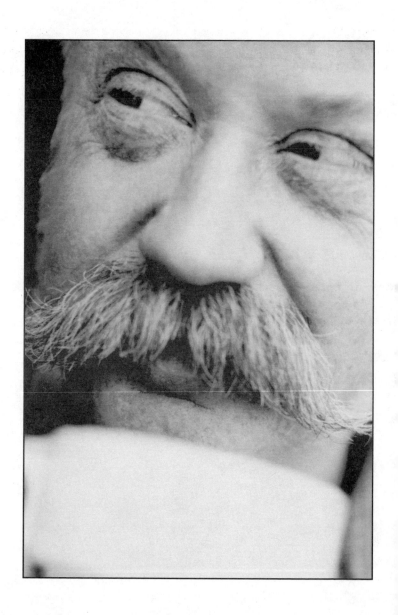

CHAPTER 8

Going the Extra Distance

I helped her with her hair. Eyebrows penciled, lipstick in place, she absolutely glowed. As I wheeled her into her husband's room, I saw him turn his gaze and attempt a smile. The paralysis slurred his words; I couldn't understand him, but she did. As I rolled her over to him, her hand reached for his and she held it to her face. It was a tearful goodbye; I saw Mr. C. mouth "I love you," and she replied the same.

—Lorraine Randall

Although nurses' resources are limited, they find a way to give communion, homemade soup, gifts, money, clothing, time, and energy. They have learned valuable lessons in their careers that many high-powered executives may never learn. They have learned that in giving you receive, in giving you are continually blessed, and in giving you garner strength to guide others.

Nurses have learned to care and feel affection for those less fortunate. They know the value of advocacy, creating options, and creating new directions. They are part of the family. After all, they care for many patients for weeks, for months, and even longer. This is why they go out of their way to pick up coffee for a grieving family member as part of their morning routine.

Nurses recognize that parents of sick children need respite, that is, a few hours away from the demands of the child on ventilation. They experience firsthand the helplessness families endure day by day because resources to help are nonexistent. If the nurse hadn't started the ball rolling, few programs would exist for children today. If the nurse didn't care, kids at home would suffer. Families with special-needs children aren't willing to leave their helpless children with strangers. The care is so technical. They need trained persons as caregivers—and these often are nurses.

Nurses who walk the extra mile know they must work harder. They can't settle for status quo. Good is not good enough, because they want more. Inquiry rules nurses' lives. Is there more to diagnoses? Is there more to discover when there is abnormal laughter, an unsteady gait, or an altered grip? Her pupils responded unequally and at different speeds; her grips, arm and leg strengths also had subtle differences. These assessments don't add up. Someone else should look at this patient.

Nurses often act on intuition. A feeling that the problem is bigger. The sense that doom is around the corner is often what forces a nurse to look further and alert others. It is hard to understand intuition. It is not learned or studied, read, or molded. It's hard to explain why additional assessments are needed, but the nurse just felt uncomfortable with what was known. It's hard to say why the order was questioned but, thankfully, the nurse wasn't satisfied. It's hard to say why you triple-checked the spelling of the medication—just a hunch that offset disaster.

Nurses are committed. They pursue what is needed regardless of whether a patient can pay or not. They stay at the patient's side; they ask critical questions. They advocate for the patient. They go beyond the present and think about the future.

LETTING THE SCRIPTURES BE THE GUIDE
by Penny Phares (Florida, USA)

It was 1984 when I met 16-year-old Jerry. I was working for Children's Medical Services in a special project. My job was to assist parents and teachers who care for handicapped children. This day I was at a special school for profoundly retarded children. Jerry's teachers were very proud of him. He had been working on holding up his head for most of the school year. If you were sent to school having cerebral palsy before the 1980s, it pretty much meant you were invisible to the world except perhaps to your parents or your teachers. Before PS94-143, when the government mandated that all of America's children would be provided an education in a least restrictive environment, children like Jerry were kept at home, out of sight, or placed in an institution, out of sight.

I was deeply affected by this handsome young man, who with his beautiful brown eyes fringed with long dark lashes looked to his teacher for praise at his efforts. His body was long and lean. He weighed about 85 pounds and was bent to one side because of scoliosis and years of no pressure on long bones, as well as muscles pulling against each other in response to jumbled neuron signals. He had a thick brown crew cut and peach fuzz that was almost a beard interspersed with adolescent acne.

It was hard for me to see past the signs of puberty until a favorite toy, a baby rattle, was placed in his hands. The teacher and the aide struggled to turn him on his back to change his diapers. The process took a while because the results of a teenage appetite, contorted contractures, and thick wiry pubic hair made it difficult. I was struck! Here is a human being who is very aware of his surroundings, obviously hears and sees and takes in information, but cannot move and cannot speak. He has the developmental level of a 3-month-old infant in the body of a teenage boy. In the coming years, he will grow larger and still need to be cared for like an infant.

When I met Jerry's family and the family of the other handicapped children in my caseload, I drove home every day in tears. These families loved their children and provided good homes and special care for them. When I asked them what I could do to help them, the repeated request was, "I wish I could find someone to help me take care of my child." These families were not willing to leave their helpless children with a stranger. Many of the relatives they trusted were afraid because the care was often very technical or the child was too fragile and might die in their care.

I covered three rural counties in Florida. Day after day I drove and cried. I was a new Christian at the time and cried and prayed, "Dear God, how can I find help for these families when there are no resources?" One morning I was reading the Bible and found a passage in Isaiah.

> Is this not the fast I have chosen; to loose the bonds of wickedness,
>
> To undo the heavy burdens, to let the oppressed go free, and to break every yoke?
>
> Is it not to share your bread with the hungry,
>
> And that you bring to your house the poor who are cast out; when you see the naked,
>
> That you cover him, and not hide yourself from your own flesh?

I had heard people say that Florence Nightingale was crazy because she heard a calling from God. I also heard that God spoke to His children through His word, but I was really unsettled about this. Was I to bring these kids to my house so their parents could have a break? But, God, I have a husband and a son and only two bedrooms!

Months went by and the problem persisted. As I traveled the roads I was convinced that God was speaking to me about providing an answer for these families, but I was afraid to tell my husband about this situation because he might think I was nuts, and then what would I do about God? So I prayed for courage to talk with him about what I thought I should do.

A few weeks later my husband attended some meetings in another county where one of my patients lived and attended the same meetings with his mother. During the meetings, the mom had her little boy, my patient Troy, back in the nursery because his breathing was so heavy and rattled. She was afraid it would disturb the assembly. Troy was her second child with Menke's Syndrome. This was a maternal genetic disease that prohibited the absorption of copper. These children have no melanin and no muscle tension. Troy was 4 years old and floppy like a rag doll, and his mother spent almost 2 hours feeding him (poor suck and swallow reflex, no head control, and multiple upper respiratory infections). Her first son died at the age of two. This mom was tired, depressed, and feeling guilty that her son was so thin. The marriage was rocky, and the older sister was lonely.

When I visited this family the following week, Troy's mother told me what a compassionate husband I had. "He was so tender when he came back to the nursery to see Troy," she said. "I have never met a man who was interested in him and would actually hold his hand."

"Are you sure it was my husband?" I asked.

She convinced me that my stoic Marine Corp-welder spouse was approachable on the subject of handicapped children, so I went to him that evening. He thought it was a great idea. He thought that instead of remodeling our own home, we should purchase the house next door to our own and make it into a four-bed retreat for children with special needs. He and another friend offered to serve on the board and establish the Isaiah Foundation, Inc. as a non-profit charitable organization to assist families with respite care. So I waited. Certainly God would provide the $150,000 to purchase and renovate this house that had been empty for so long. The owners were eager to sell it. They lived in another state and had no intention of returning to the house. I went to work with plans and ideas about a Hubbard tank and an arboretum with birds and butterflies and sensory stimulation. My husband started the ball rolling to get fire permits and zoning adjustments. Two years went by. The house remained empty.

When the mayor of the town got wind of the project, he began a campaign to prohibit the initiation of any kind of facility that would change the climate of the neighborhood. The battle that ensued was confusing to me. How could a home for children who could not speak and could not move lead to a town full of halfway houses for drug addicts?

In October 1989 the state of Florida passed a law that provided for group homes and foster facilities of up to eight residents to be allowed in residential neighborhoods, regardless of local zoning. In November the house next door sold to someone else. I had the distinct impression that God was chuckling at my assumptions.

In the meantime, the situation for Troy's family became worse, and we started taking care of this child in our home on the weekends to give his parents a break. The very difficult task of feeding, diapering, suctioning, and watching the clear blue eyes of this sweet face as he worked to draw each breath and swallow each bite was overwhelming. What if this were my child? What if I had to do these tasks and feel these emotions 24 hours a day every day of the week—for years?

Troy's plight became public and others in the community came forward to expand the board of directors of the Isaiah Foundation. These men and women suggested a needs assessment. How many families are there who need respite care? Over the next few months we solicited input from families in school systems, social services, and healthcare agencies in 16 counties. The response enabled us to hear from actual families. We learned that at that time in 1989, there were about 350 families who would benefit from respite care within 60 miles of the facility we planned. It was pretty apparent to me that we would not be able to serve them in a four-bed facility for very long. The board of directors recommended that we train care givers to go to the families and care for the children in their own homes.

That was the last thing this nurse wanted to do. How could I train lay people to go into a situation where I had no control over their performance? What about my own professional license? Yet within a week, I was invited to participate in a training-for-trainers of the FDLRS (Florida Diagnostic and Learning Resource Services) MITCH (Models for Interdisciplinary Training for Children with Handicaps) program. Parents were not professionals, yet they learned about positioning and feeding, and suctioning and seizure control. I found we could do this!

Parents could be introduced to individuals who were compassionate and caring and who were trained to care for the special needs of their kids. Parents would take responsibility for completing the training of the care giver for their particular child and determine if they would leave their child with the care giver. The Isaiah Foundation would do the training, provide background checks, and subsidize the cost of the care if it were beyond the parents' means. In 1992 the Isaiah Foundation held its first training course and began providing care in five counties.

Jerry and Troy and many others have passed on. They have taught us so much about patience and kindness and quality of life. After 20 years of "corporate" respectability, I know that it is nursing that drove my desire to pursue this activity, because I remembered to ALWAYS be FAMILY DRIVEN.

The Florida Board of Nursing approved the training course. Nurses capable of teaching appeared out of nowhere (a real miracle when you consider the nursing shortage). One county has become so actively involved in the work of the weak and disabled that it became an independent agency. Laws have changed since 1984, and organizations like Fundamentally for Families, the Bureau of Exceptional Education, PS94-457 Part B, and the Medicaid Waiver Program have improved the situation for disabled children in Florida. As nurses we know that our perspective always leaves us with the feeling that more needs to be done and things move too slowly, but the promise is at the end of the verse in Isaiah:

> Then your light shall break forth like the morning, your healing shall spring forth speedily. If you extend your soul to the hungry and satisfy the afflicted soul, then your light shall dawn in the darkness and your darkness shall be as the noon day. (Isaiah 58:8, 10)

ACTING AS THE SPOKESPERSON AND ADVOCATE
by Roberta Jerz (Florida, USA)

Father B was a frail, cachectic, 85-year-old Roman Catholic priest who had given nearly 50 years of his life to serve God and others. He moved to South Fort Myers from a small town in Connecticut. It was in this small town that he built a beautiful church where he pastored for many years before retiring for health reasons. When Fr. B was not visiting the sick or ministering to the bereaved, he could be found mowing the grass in the summer, or cleaning the parking lot of snow in the winter. For Fr. B, being a good steward meant doing activities above and beyond his priestly duties.

In Florida, Fr. B lived in a cramped, one-bedroom travel trailer. He would sometimes bump his head on the door frame, because he was a lanky 6 ft. 3 in. and weighed about 150 pounds. He was oxygen-dependent as his body was ravaged by the effects of end-stage emphysema. He had difficulty breathing on exertion, but this did not stop him from getting into his car and going shopping for his humble needs or making his frequent doctor appointments, always carrying a portable oxygen tank.

Fr. B's neighbors always smiled and waved as he drove by. They frequently offered their help, which he sometimes accepted. Carrying groceries was one of his biggest challenges. One friendly couple told him about a parish nurse (me) who worked at the nearby Catholic church and made home visits. Since he did not attend Mass at the nearby Catholic church where I worked, I was pleased when he called me to make a home visit. During my initial visit with Fr. B, I discovered he had just spent more than $280 on medications that his personal health insurance would have paid for. He told me, "I felt hurried as I fumbled through all of these cards in my wallet so I just paid cash!" After Fr. B gave me permission to recover the medication costs, I placed a call to his insurance company. After explaining the situation to them, they set up a conference call that included the pharmacy, the insurance company, and me. We received immediate satisfaction! A check would be sent out the next day for a full reimbursement

After that initial incident, I visited Fr. B weekly. His openness and friendliness made it possible for us to discover everything from music and medical problems to emotional needs and the end of life. He told me about his living will and of the person who had his power of attorney, who lived nearby but was vacationing out of the country at that time. He also talked about his beloved niece. She was one of three living relatives left in his family, who called him from Connecticut every day to check on him. He shared stories about his family.

One day he asked me if I would give him Holy Communion. This to me was quite an honor because I knew that he celebrated Mass privately on his own every morning. In his home he kept a supply of "hosts" (the Holy Communion wafers, which in the Catholic faith, literally means the body of Christ). We grew to be close friends and I looked forward to our visits. Often I brought homemade soup from a lady in our church who was not only a great cook but also one of my volunteer parish nurses. In turn, Fr. B enjoyed making me copies of his extensive collection of cassette tapes—mostly classical and easy listening. He wanted me to listen and enjoy his music as I rode around in my car making home visits. He was that kind of man!

One day he traveled, unbeknownst to me, to the store, and dragged along his oxygen tank. He purchased bags of candy and plastic containers so he could fill them and give them to me to deliver to shut-ins. "Everyone needs a little chocolate," he said.

Fr. B was not a healthy man. He suffered from severe gastric distress along with dyspnea. He took many medications including prednisone that may have contributed to his abdominal pain. On a scale of 1-10 he would rate the pain at a 10 plus. There were times when the pain would double him over and bring tears to his eyes. With his permission, I called his doctor, made an appointment, and arranged transportation with a close neighbor. I wrote down pertinent information along with a current list of his medications, which he agreed to share with the doctor. As Fr. B was a private person, he refused my offer to accompany him.

I continued to visit and teach about nutrition and pain issues. I worried about his anorexia as I watched his gaunt frame lose more weight. Hopefully he would eat some of the soup that I brought him each visit. One afternoon he called me at home. I went to him immediately, and after a quick assessment, I took him to the nearby hospital emergency department. Tests were run and to my surprise, he was sent home with another prescription in hand! Another medication to attempt to quiet his agonizing pain—but what was its source?

Shortly after returning from the hospital, Fr. B phoned again. His voice was glazed with pain, and I heard his desperate anguish. "I'm so sorry to bother you again but I need you to come. I can't even get out of bed. It feels like I am being stuck with knives in my abdomen!" I asked, "Do you need an ambulance?" "No—just come," he quietly pleaded.

Immediately my husband (a policeman) and I drove across town to Fr. B's side. I quickly assessed him and determined that we needed EMS and called 911. Within 5 minutes EMS arrived taking Fr. B back to the hospital. As he laid in the stark emergency department, I noted his modesty and asked my husband to help him undress. Fr. B thankfully accepted. He handed me his keys and wallet for safekeeping and was soon whisked off for x-rays. We stayed until we were assured by the doctor that he would be admitted to receive the help he so desperately needed.

The test revealed Fr. B. had a large tumor. It was abscessed and pressing against his pancreas causing intense pain. Surgery was needed as soon as possible, and again, I talked to Fr. B about the issue of a living will. He was clear in stating he did not want to be hooked up to a respirator if it was discovered that he was in a terminal state with no chance for recovery. Surgery was performed the next day, which led to the diagnosis of advanced cancer of the pancreas. The surgeon stated, "The tumor was so large we could not get it all, and it has metastasized. It was the abscess that caused all of this pain." I visited Fr. B as he lay in the ICU intubated and in pain as evidenced by his furrowed brow and the deep facial grimace. I stopped by the nurses station and asked them to give him pain medication. The nurse replied, "He was recently medicated with morphine 2 mg ... it's not quite time yet!" I then inquired about Fr. B's living will. No copy was found on his chart despite several hospital admissions in the past.

Unable to contact the person who had Fr. B's power of attorney, I placed a call to Fr. B's niece in Connecticut. I asked her to fax a copy of his living will to me as soon as possible and to come to Fort Myers to be an advocate for her beloved uncle. "But he is improving—the doctor called me and told me that!" she exclaimed. I again said, "Please come anyway. I have worked with hospice and dying patients for several years now, and I believe Fr. B hasn't long to live." I received a faxed copy of the living will right away and had it placed on the front of his chart. I then contacted hospice to make a referral. Within 2 days his niece arrived and Fr. B was admitted to hospice. "I am so glad I listened to you and came right away," she cried. "I might not have seen him alive if I had waited."

The last day I saw Fr. B alive was again in the ICU. He was very much aware of my presence. His eyes looked into mine with a softened friendship. My eyes were full of tears and my throat felt closed with emotion. "I love you, Fr. B," I whispered. He smiled and squeezed my hand and attempted to whisper, "I love you, too." I thanked him for the honor of just knowing him and allowing me into his world. And he just smiled in an all-knowing way.

Later that day, Fr. B was transferred to a hospice house by non-emergency transport. He died very peacefully the next day with a Catholic priest and a male nurse at his side. I came in right after his passing and could not stop the tears. Tears for myself because a gentle soul had left my physical sight and tears for the suffering that he had to endure in his last days of life. I left with a heavy heart.

The next month I received a surprise letter in my mailbox. It was a letter from Fr. B's niece. She had also enclosed a special gift. It was his rosary. She thought it would be meaningful to me. I will always cherish that gift, as I cherish Fr. B's memory. This is what parish nursing is all about.

PROVIDING UNEXPECTED RESOURCES
by Susan Whatley (Florida, USA)

I am a certified trauma and emergency care nurse for children, which allows me to be part of the trauma team within the emergency department. This means if a trauma patient comes in, I would be the primary nurse to care for that patient. The trauma nurse takes care of the patient until a final disposition is made, such as the patient is to be admitted, go to surgery, be transferred to another facility for further care, or sometimes go to the morgue. I love doing trauma nursing because I can see immediate outcomes with each nursing intervention.

During one particular shift, I was reminded what nursing is truly all about. My day had been going well, in fact, it was almost half over and we hadn't had one trauma. I was thinking about being able to go home and put up my feet. I had seen the routine patients that day: cold symptoms, lacerations, a patient threatening suicide. I was just glad the department wasn't overflowing with patients because I was almost 7 months pregnant with my fourth child, and I was tired!

The phone rang, one long, distinctive ring—our dedicated direct line from emergency dispatch. That meant a trauma was being called in from the field. My heart sank when I heard it was a 9-month-old baby girl burned in a fire, with burns on her face, arm, and leg. The paramedics reported she was maintaining an open airway on her own.

With an estimated arrival time of 15 minutes, we went into action getting equipment ready for an infant: setting up the cardiac monitor, pulling out warmed IV fluids, and preparing the pediatric resuscitation cart should it be needed. All the support staff started arriving: people from surgery, anesthesia, radiology, and social work, and the trauma surgeon.

A few minutes later, the helicopter landed outside and our little patient was brought in. The paramedics told us Baby E. was in her crib in a back bedroom of her mobile home when a faulty light above her bed shorted and caused a fire. Her mother had rushed in and got her and her two siblings out. The house was gutted. Baby E. had approximately 12 to 14% total burns to her face, right arm, and right leg. She was alert and crying, which in this case was a good sign. It meant she had an open airway.

As I worked quickly to establish an IV, to administer pain medication and fluids, I noticed her tracking me with her eyes, watching every move I made. I talked to her in soothing tones and stroked the arm that was unburned even though I longed to pick her up and hold her, to comfort her. I was told her mother was on the way. Her other children were getting examined at another area hospital.

After receiving some pain medicine and having her burns dressed, Baby E. quieted down and appeared interested in all that was going on around her. Even though she was more comfortable and relaxed, I stayed alert for any potential changes in her pulmonary status, knowing that burn victims can rapidly develop respiratory distress. If Baby E. were to go into distress, she would have to be intubated immediately.

The social worker brought Baby E.'s mother in as soon as she arrived at the hospital. She was frightened and tearful, even more so because she spoke no English, only Spanish. No matter how well we try to prepare families and loved ones for what they'll see when they enter that trauma room, it just doesn't compare with the reality of the sights and sounds of what is happening: the monitors, the alarms, the rush of people, seeing someone they love in the midst of it all.

I asked the social worker, who spoke Spanish, to tell the mother her daughter was okay. I also told her I had given her daughter some medicine for pain and tended to the burns, and that she would need to be

transferred to a burn center for additional care. I further explained tha
Baby E. would be cared for by doctors and nurses whose specialty i
children with burns. She nodded her head with understanding an
appeared almost immediately relieved.

The trauma surgeon spoke with a physician in Cincinnati, and th
decision was made to transfer her to the Shriner's Children's Hospita
as soon as possible. The social worker started making arrangement
with the local Shriners. They would pay for a plane ticket for th
patient and her mom on the next available commercial flight. A Shrine
was on his way to pick up the tickets and would bring them right t
the hospital.

As I made the necessary arrangements on my end, including callin
report to the nurse who would be taking over her care and makin
copies of all the lab and radiology reports, I began thinking about th
hardships that Baby E. and her mom would be facing. Not only woul
the mother have her hands full with a burned baby for hours befor
getting to the hospital; they would be going to a strange place. Th
mother would have no way to communicate with anyone unless the
spoke Spanish. I worried about her and the baby going on the plane
being in another city so far from home and being all on their own unti
the baby was well enough to come home. We had treated the patient
arrangements were in the works to transport her, and relatives woul
care for the other children. Everyone had done what was required
However, I knew it wasn't going to be enough.

I looked down at the small plastic bag with the Wal-Mart logo tha
Mom had brought with her. It was all she had in the world now, every
thing that they had owned was gone. She had managed to salvage a few
changes of clothes for herself. That was it. I got on the phone and calle
the Infant Care Center across the street, the day care that I would be
taking my baby to after I came back from maternity leave. I explaine

hat I had a pediatric patient with no clothes who was going to be transerred out of state. I asked them if they happened to have a baby gown hey could spare for her and they started looking. I sent a technician ›ver to get it. I gave Baby E. some more pain medication and checked ıer vital signs. She was continuing to do well; her respirations remained :asy with clear lung sounds, and her dressings remained clean and dry. gave mom some juice and crackers; I was sure she hadn't had a thing o eat all day.

I found out, after talking further with Baby E.'s mother (through ınother interpreter), that she only had 30 cents with her and not much nore in the bank. There was no way I was letting this woman go with›ut even enough money to buy a can of soda. I had 4 dollars in my pock-:t, my lunch money. Four dollars wasn't going to be that much help. She vould need more than that. I walked out into the hallway and asked the irst staff member I saw, "Did you have lunch yet?" He replied, "No." I said n my most assertive voice, "Good, give me your lunch money, I need it." went on to the next person, and the next. People were cheerfully ıanding over their money. I had more than $60 within a few minutes! Not bad for so little time! I'd gotten Mom a snack, some money, and a ;own for the baby; now she would need something written in English, o others could help her find her way.

I sat down and wrote a quick note, explaining the baby had burns, so he airline staff would take special care of them. I wrote the flight num›er, airline, and destination in detail in the event she got lost. She would ›e able to show this letter to anyone and they would be able to direct ıer. It would also aid the Shriner picking her up at the airport in Cincinnati. I asked the doctor to give me a verbal order so I could also ,end a dose of pain medicine with Mom to give the baby by mouth, if ıeed be. I got baby bottles of formula and diapers to send. In a short vhile, the Shriner came to get them; Mom gave me a long bear hug and kissed my cheek (I didn't need a translator for that—some things are universal).

As I sit here writing this, my new little son is playing quietly with his toes, as all is right with his world. I'm so thankful that I could use everything I've ever learned in nursing to take a bad situation and make it right. As nurses, we can be proud of our skills, our competence, and our compassion. That is what makes the difference of merely going through the motions of caring for patients and making things right with their world. That is what makes us nurses.

Taking a bad situation and making it right, righting certain wrongs in this world, and making sure the patient comes first are the ways nurses go the extra distance. So often nurses care for patients who are so "down on luck." So often they care for the poor, the lonely, and those with few resources. The nurses in these stories are not wealthy people in the dollar sense of the word, but wealthy in giving. They care about others. This is unconditional caring. Taking a few moments to look at the whole picture, being unique in knowing that there is an underlying problem, scratching beneath the surface, and knowing that if you keep true to yourself you can uncover mysteries that others may not see.

NOT LETTING THE PATIENT "SHUT HER OUT"
by Lorraine Randall (Florida, USA)

It was the beginning of my 12-hour shift. I had been off for 3 days and would undoubtedly receive a different group of patients. Usually this is rue, but my patients tend to have much longer stays due to multiple, often-complicated morbidities. During shift-to-shift report, I learned about the patient in 424, Evelyn C. She was a 70-something-year-old woman who was admitted with pneumonia and failure to thrive. She had a history of cardiopulmonary disease (COPD) and cardiovascular accident (CVA) with associated upper extremity, left-sided weakness and flaccidity of the lower extremities, leaving her essentially wheelchair bound. I asked if there was family and what the long-term plans were. There was a family but no one knew much about them. Discharge plans had not been made. The night nurse proceeded to warn me the patient was an angry woman who could not be pleased.

I made my rounds going from room to room. Finally I arrived at 424. I tapped lightly on the door and was promptly told by a faceless voice to go away. I explained to the voice in the dark that I was her nurse and asked if I could come in. Surprisingly she granted permission. I entered the room and turned on the light, surveying the person in the bed. Evelyn, all of maybe 100 pounds was pale and fragile looking. She had soft, wavy wheat-colored hair, with furrowing eyebrows above eyes that scornfully surveyed me. "Well, whatever it is you want, do it and get out of here," she said. I remember thinking to myself, oh boy, do I have my work cut out for me today. I did an assessment but began to get this nagging feeling. There was something so familiar about this woman, but I couldn't put my finger on it. Every time I thought I might remember, Evelyn would yell at me. She didn't speak, she yelled short commands, and would answer in a short, snappy way. Instinctively, intuitively, I knew there was a lot going on here. Unfortunately there were many demands at that particular time of day, so it was not the right time to pursue the source of Evelyn's anger.

It was one o'clock in the afternoon, while I was passing out medications, when I returned to Evelyn's room. She was in the bed having refused to get up to the chair for lunch. Her over-bed table held a untouched lunch tray. I asked her if the food was not good or if she di not have an appetite. She merely told me to take the tray away. removed the tray and handed her a cup with her medication in it. Sh told me to take it away, also.

I think one of the hardest things to cope with in nursing is being th target of someone's misplaced anger. It is almost an instinctive, guttu al reflex to react, not always in a positive manner, even though inte lectually you know that it is not you personally. It is just that you ar there. It is easy to do just what she wants and go away. However, I an not a quitter. So I said, "You can send me away now but I promise yo I'll be back. Okay, you don't have to take the medication now but I' bring it back in an hour."

For such a little woman with such respiratory problems, she sur could yell. And it worried me to see her exert herself this way. Evely proceeded to tell me that I had "some nerve" and "who did I think was, I didn't care about her" and "probably wouldn't care if sh dropped dead tomorrow."

After this response, I pulled a chair over to the bedside, sat, and qui etly waited until she was finished. For a short period of time, we jus looked at each other; I used this time to gather my thoughts and pos my next statements so as not to further agitate her. I said, "Evelyn, it' quite evident that you are in a tremendous amount of pain. I know yo don't know me, or for that matter trust me, but I am here for you. Pleas tell me why you hurt so badly. I don't know if I can help but sometime it just helps to talk."

Evelyn stared at me incredulously, and I waited for another tongu lashing, but instead she broke down and began to sob loudly. Throug the sobs she began her story. As I listened to her speak, that sense o familiarity returned, and then I remembered why.

Evelyn's husband had been diagnosed some 5 or 6 years ago with a rare neurological disorder called para supra nuclear palsy (PSP). Mr. C. had actually been a patient on our unit. I now remember caring for him. Evelyn doesn't remember me, as that time of her life she said was "blur." As she continued to speak, the memories returned, and quite vividly, because this was only the second patient I cared for with PSP. It was very traumatic for the family, and they did not take the news well. They had actually arranged to transfer the patient to a facility up north where research regarding the disease was being done. As it turned out, the diagnosis was confirmed and the patient eventually returned home.

Evelyn assumed the care giver role. At first she said it wasn't too bad. Actually she said anything she could do that would keep her husband of some 50 years with her was worth it. But the toll of being the sole care giver wore heavily on her, as we have all witnessed to be the case of care givers. Three years ago she had a devastating stroke. She had to go to rehabilitation. Her only child, a son, lived in the area, but she said he was a busy family man and had to work. Plus, his wife was "a bit hard to take."

Evelyn said her son had no choice but to place Mr. C. in the nursing home. When Evelyn finally was released from rehabilitation, she was no longer able to care for her beloved husband. She not only couldn't care for him, but she also had to rely on her son to take her to visit Mr. C. in the nursing home. Because of her son's schedule, she would sometimes go 2 weeks without seeing her spouse. "It broke my heart," she said. "The short time we had left I couldn't even spend with him." Evelyn then proceeded to tell me about the endless number of aides who would come to the house two to three times a week to help her shower, etc. Basically she described an existence of dependence, a life almost totally confined to her condo, with only those brief visits to Mr. C. to look forward to.

As I thought back and remembered the wife of my patient all thos years ago, I remembered a fiercely robust woman who would no could not, accept what the neurologist had to offer. She was a fighter, force to be reckoned with. But things had changed.

"How is your husband doing?" I asked. "He's here in the hospital," sh told me. Then she told me that Mr. C. had been admitted about 5 day ago with complications of his disease. "Where is he? Have you see him?" She told me she had not seen him in 3 weeks, which has bee very hard to accept. But her son "keeps me informed," she said. I coul n't believe this. Husband and wife are in the same hospital and haven seen each other! That was not a good thing.

Well, I needed to take one issue at a time. First I needed to locate M C. and find out about his condition. Then I needed to get the soci worker to devise a plan that was better for both patients. There had t be a way for this woman to see her husband more frequently! As I tol her that and started for the door, I met her son coming in. I asked hi what room his father was in. I could not believe the answer. He said h dad was in room 416, only a few doors away! Evelyn had been in tl hospital 1 week and her husband 5 days, and neither had seen the othe She had every right in the world to be furious, I would have been too.

When I checked on Mr. C's condition, he was doing okay. He was be discharged back to the nursing home a few days later. I spoke to h nurse and arranged for husband and wife to have dinner together th night. I went back to Evelyn's room and told her I wanted her to g some rest because she was having dinner with her husband. Her fac lit up and for the first time that day I saw a smile.

I placed a call to the medical social worker and discussed the fam ly situation. I knew there were facilities in our area that could probab accommodate both patients' needs and keep them together. The soci worker agreed and promised to talk to Evelyn that afternoon.

Dinnertime arrived. I helped Mr. C's nurse get him into the chair. He could still feed himself once his plate and food were properly arranged. I arranged for a wheelchair with an oxygen tank for Evelyn. I helped her with her hair. With her eyebrows penciled, lipstick in place, she absolutely glowed. As I wheeled her into her husband's room, I saw him turn his gaze and attempt a smile. The paralysis slurred his words. I couldn't understand him, but she did. As I rolled her over to him, her hand reached for his and she held it to her face. I set up the trays and gave them their much-needed privacy. After awhile it was time for Evelyn to go back to her room. It was a tearful goodbye. I saw Mr. C. mouth "I love you" and she replied the same. I realized the two probably thought it would be weeks before they saw each other again. So I said, "Evelyn, you have every right to see your husband anytime you want while you are both here. You just let someone know you want to come over and I promise you it will happen." And I made sure this promise would be kept. I spoke to my resource person. On a busy unit, it's easy to understand how this oversight might have occurred. But the word was out now, and it was agreed the couple would share at least one meal a day together. And do you know what? Evelyn ate

The medical social worker did get together with Evelyn. She was given information about a local facility that offered two levels of care. One was assisted living, which meant Evelyn could have her privacy but get help when she needed it. She could also surround herself with her precious belongings. Mr. C. would have skilled nursing care. The best news of all was they would be able to see each other anytime they desired. The paperwork was submitted and it was a done deal. How wonderful for them both! It was amazing to see Evelyn transformed from her previous state to the grinning person I found in the bed the next morning. She told me she actually felt like she had something to look forward to. I wasn't there when she was discharged, but I was told all went well and the couple was together at last.

This had to be one of the easiest interventions I've ever done, but I really do believe the effects of this simple intervention affected two lives tremendously. I'm so glad I didn't let Evelyn shut me out.

EXTENDING CARE TO THE FAMILY
by Caryl Wheeler (Florida, USA)

On a March evening while listening to the local news, my ears perked up as the anchorwoman spoke of a man in critical condition at Tampa General Hospital. The newsperson recounted how the patient had contracted hepatitis A from a salad served by a caterer at a church picnic. His illness had progressed in a rapid downward spiral, and he had just received a liver transplant as a consequence.

As I watched this news story, I remember thinking how serendipitous life is, and although all liver transplant patients are critical the first day, most do well postoperatively. However, his post-surgical condition was certainly not atypical, and I assumed a probable normal course of recovery was in his future. Little did I know Mr. M would be assigned as my patient the next day and that his treatment would be long and arduous. Because of my experience with him and his family, my personal and professional lives were about to change forever.

The next morning I received report and had my first formal introduction to Mr. M's case. As I walked into his room to conduct the first morning assessment, I was struck by all the family photos that surrounded him. My first impression was that someone certainly cared about this man.

Familiarizing myself with his history, I noted Mr. M was 46 years old and had been in good health before contracting hepatitis. Prior to transplant, his medical condition had become critical. The liver transplant had been essential to continued life. His kidneys were beginning to fail, and Mr. M had been placed on dialysis therapy. His prognosis was unclear.

Proceeding with his assessment, I was soon interrupted by a call. It was Mr. M's wife. She wanted to visit. Regular unit visiting hours are 9 a.m. to 9 p.m. I noted it was only 8 a.m., but knowing her presence would not hinder my care giving or negatively impact Mr. M's rest, I invited Mrs. M to come back to his room. Mrs. M. would become a fixture at his bedside, and I soon enlisted her as a partner and ally in the delivery of his care. This relationship was to extend over many months.

As time went by, Mr. M's condition slowly deteriorated. He developed respiratory failure and was unable to be weaned from mechanical ventilation. Eventually a tracheotomy was ordered.

I recall his wife expressing concern at the time about how the procedure might affect Mr. M's ability to sing. I explained to her that having a tracheotomy would help in the process of weaning her husband from the ventilator. At the time, I was thinking of Mr. M. as a liver transplant. I did not associate Mrs. M's concern for his singing voice with Mr. M, the person and personality. Only later did the importance of this statement become clear.

Days passed and turned to weeks and eventually months of intensive care. Mr. M valiantly struggled but remained gravely ill. The presence of his wife and family, constant and stalwart, had become commonplace, and I knew their bedside watch was emotionally draining. As I cared for Mr. M, I exchanged daily conversation with his family and was taken by how kind and considerate they were to the medical team. They were as concerned for us as care givers as they were for Mr. M and his progress.

As I was leaving work one afternoon, I reflected on Mr. M's difficult course and the relationship I had developed with him. It was then that I realized as I had cared for Mr. M. and watched him lose ground day-by-day, I had come to know his case thoroughly but had not really gotten to know him as an individual. Instead, it was his wife, sons, daughters-in-law, and minister I had gotten to know, and through them I had learned about Mr. M.

Mrs. M was a pillar of strength, spending most of each day with her husband. Knowing this, I often brought her coffee as part of my morning routine. I had developed a special relationship with this family and felt they had become not only collaborators in the care of Mr. M., but also my support system.

The days progressed and it seemed I was with Mr. M as often as his family. Mrs. M commented on this and said that she believed I must have to work every holiday—I had cared for Mr. M. on Easter, Mother's Day, and Memorial Day. On Father's Day, I observed Mrs. M crying at his bedside. She said she was having a weak moment. As she shared her concern, we hugged. This event made me realize that I had been welcomed into her emotional inner circle.

At the end of June, the staff learned Mr. M's prognosis had become terminal. By the second week of July, it was evident the time had been reached for a decision with the family regarding Mr. M's end-of-life care. After discussing this need with co-workers, we arranged a family conference for Mrs. M with Mr. M's primary physician, Dr. B.

I was not scheduled to work the day of the conference but thought I was needed there, as I had developed a deep concern for the family. Knowing the conference would be an emotionally difficult experience, I drove to the meeting. After the conference was over, I was relieved. Dr. B did an excellent job in explaining Mr. M's deteriorating condition and the little hope that remained. I was glad I had attended. Mrs. M and the family asked me and Dr. B to stay while they discussed Mr. M's situation and the difficult alternatives they faced.

They asked me to share my opinion—what would I do? I suggested Mr. M be given a "do not resuscitate" (DNR) status and I shared my reasons. Mrs. M was uncomfortable doing this. She was not yet ready to accept Mr. M's impending death. After the family conference, another nurse and I spoke with Dr. B about our thoughts. Mrs. M considered the options we had discussed and ultimately decided to slowly withdraw care. Upon reflection, she accepted the fact that a DNR status was in Mr. M's best interest and shared her thoughts with his physician. Dr. B wrote the DNR orders. A few days later, Mr. M died.

Because of my relationship with Mr. M, through his family, I felt compelled to attend his funeral. It was at the funeral that I learned how central he had been to his family unit and the community in which he lived. In the eulogy, his minister reviewed his life. He spoke of a man who loved his family and God. Mr. M loved music; he toured and sang with a band. He was proud of the fact that he had sung at the Grand Ole Opry and was the music director at his church. No wonder his wife had been concerned about his tracheotomy and the impact on his singing abilities!

The minister revealed that only those in his hometown knew of him until he contracted hepatitis, had a liver transplant, and died. Now, the whole country knew his name. The minister helped the family accept his passing and while doing so, reached out and gave praise to the nursing staff who had cared for Mr. M throughout his illness.

It was not until the funeral that I realized how much I had cared for Mr. M's family over the preceding months and, in turn, how much care and support I had received from them.

When nurses provide attention to the patient and family alike, they not only care for the emotional well-being of the patients but, in turn, receive mutual support from the community of family and visitors. The impact of this service multiplies our value and effectiveness as care givers and, in turn, increases job satisfaction exponentially.

INTERVENING AT CRITICAL TIMES
by Sheila Ferrall (Florida, USA)

> Behold, I'm going to send an angel before you to guide you along the way. Exodus 23:20.

Those were the words painstakingly cross-stitched on the beautifully framed piece that Amy gave me on her last visit. We had grown close over that year. And now her treatment was finished, and she was moving away.

I'll never forget our first meeting. I walked into the examination room and introduced myself to the young couple there. She was 28 years old and her husband was about the same age. She looked like a typical, fit, healthy young woman. The only clue something was amiss was the stylish turban she wore on her head to cover a recent surgical site. In the span of only a couple of weeks, she had learned she had a brain tumor and had surgery for its removal. She was sure it was a death sentence. I can only describe her behavior on that first visit as my grandmother would—"she was fidgety." She was in and out of her chair, pacing around the small exam room, and her eyes darted about and were often tearful. Who wouldn't be fidgety in the same situation? Amy had only been married a couple of years. Her husband served in the armed forces, and her biggest concern, up to that point in her life, had been where they would be stationed next. Suddenly, she was faced with a life-threatening diagnosis of brain tumor and the prospect of a lengthy treatment.

It was a Saturday evening like any other when Amy first had a seizure. She lost consciousness and was taken to the emergency department (ED). Extensive diagnostic tests revealed the tumor, and she was rushed to surgery. She was referred to our facility for further treatment. I sat close to her, our knees almost touching, and began my assessment. I said, in my most calm and reassuring voice, "I've been looking through your records, and it looks like you've been through a lot in the past few weeks. How are you holding up?" She cried as she shared her story and her concerns. Her husband held her hand while she spoke and his eyes mirrored her fear.

When she finished, I said, "I can only imagine how difficult the past couple of weeks have been for you. I want you to know you have come to the right place. In the overall spectrum of cancer, primary brain tumors are rare, making up about only 1-2% of all cancers. But we see and treat patients with your type of tumor all the time." I asked what she knew about chemotherapy. I always want to know about any preconceived ideas so I can address them early. "Yes," I told them, "there are side effects, and some can be pretty scary. But we are much better about anticipating and treating those side effects today than we were years ago."

The physician I work with speaks with a heavy accent, so I was worried he would be difficult to understand, particularly with their heightened anxiety. I stayed with Amy and her husband throughout that first visit. I wanted to hear the treatment plan so I'd be able to follow up with appropriate teaching. Amy was going to receive four courses of chemotherapy followed by radiation therapy. There was so much to learn. The litany of topics included chemotherapy schedules and side effects, symptom management, long-term effects, seizure precautions, and more. You can't imagine how devastating it is for a young, active, and independent woman to be told she cannot drive because of her

history of seizures and the potential for more. Suddenly, she was totally dependent on others for transportation. It did not matter that she felt
well enough to drive; she was prohibited from driving because of the
seizures. Talk about adding insult to injury. In Amy's case, her husband
was often sent away, as part of his work, and spent weeks at a time away
from home on assignment. Further, Amy wasn't from this area and her
family lived elsewhere. The next several months proved to be particularly challenging. Her chemotherapy consisted of two oral medications
and twice-a-month injections. Amy lived about 45 minutes from our
facility, so I arranged for her to get her regular lab work done closer to
her home. She had to come in for the chemotherapy injections and to
be examined, so I scheduled all other appointments around those visits. When her husband was away, her mother would sometimes fly
down from Michigan to accompany her; sometimes a friend would
bring her to the clinic for the injections. She called me often between
visits for a little "therapy." Therapy usually consisted of her relaying her
fears and concerns and me reassuring her that things were progressing
as expected. For her final course of chemotherapy, Amy asked if she
could get her last chemotherapy injection in Michigan. She had grown
weary of the hassles of treatment and wanted to be with her parents.
After several phone calls, the arrangements were made. Overall, Amy
tolerated her chemotherapy beautifully. Nausea was held at bay with an
antiemetic protocol. While her blood counts dropped with each treatment, they were never dangerously low. Amy's experience might have
been characterized as perfect if it hadn't been for reoccurring seizures.
Just when she had been seizure free for several months and thought
she might be able to drive again, she would have another episode,
requiring yet another adjustment in medications and a resetting of the
clock before she could drive again.

Amy finally finished the chemotherapy and was ready to begin radiation. However, her insurance company required she receive the radiation at a different facility. She wasn't enamored by this idea because she felt comfortable with our team. I reassured her that we weren't abandoning her and would still be available if she needed us. We would assume her follow-up after radiation was complete. During her fourth week of radiation therapy, I received a frantic phone call from Amy. I was worried that she'd had another seizure, but this time her problem was different. She reported feeling "wobbly," almost as if she were drunk. She had been to see the radiation oncologist and was started on steroids but with no real improvement in her symptoms. Amy knew the side effects from radiation to the brain are usually managed successfully with steroids. She was scared. It occurred to me that while Amy's seizures had improved, overall she seemed to be declining. I asked Amy when the last Dilantin level had been checked. She couldn't remember a check being done since starting the radiation. After consulting with her physician, I arranged for an immediate blood check of the Dilantin level, which indicated it was well over the therapeutic limit; she was experiencing toxic side effects! A simple medication adjustment and her symptoms disappeared.

We continued to follow Amy closely in the weeks after she finished therapy. She began to look forward to the future. She asked questions about starting a family. Amy was well aware of the possibility of infertility as a result of the treatment. She knew that pregnancy wasn't advised for the first 2 years after finishing therapy but wanted to be "ready" when that time period had passed. I gave her a book about sexuality and fertility after cancer treatment and made arrangements for her to have a gynecologic evaluation.

Amy's husband was transferred to a base in the northeast. I made phone calls and sent her records to a neuro-oncologist near her new home. Every Christmas I get a card and a note from Amy and her husband. The first card came with a picture of the two of them near their Christmas tree. The second year, the card included a picture of Amy, her husband, and her dog. The letters always ended the same way, always with a thank you. This year, she wrote:

"I had my most recent MRI about a week ago and there was no change. So now it is 6 years and two healthy children later. In the beginning, I found it hard to see this far ahead. Just wanted to take this opportunity to say thank you again."

Thank you, Amy. Not every story of a patient with a brain tumor has such a happy ending. My 30-year-old nephew's didn't. My dear friend and mentor's didn't. But Amy's did, and I revel in it. I take delight in it. I was part of it.

Nurses are part of the family. They often spend every holiday with these families trying to make the awful better. They go above and beyond, coming into work even on days off just to check on "things." They are simply there. Births, wakes, funerals, in the home and hospital, whenever, wherever, the nurse is there. He or she may not always be in the forefront, but that is nursing: they are behind the scenes, hoping and praying that the family, the child, the baby with a birth defect totally alone and abandoned, receives peace, love, tender human touch. Most of all, nurses, who walk the extra mile, never underestimate the power of love.

HAVING FAITH IN THE POWER OF LOVE
by Kathey Milligan (Florida, USA)

The day began, much as any other, with the usual hum in the neonatal intensive care unit (NICU). Report had barely concluded when we received a call from labor and delivery for an immediate cesarean section. The mother's history was very sketchy.

I headed immediately to the operating room (OR) knowing the neonatologist would not likely arrive before the baby would be delivered. The OR was in full swing. Everybody was moving fast. The mother's heart tones were down, and there was no time to waste. Mom was under general anesthesia. As the incision was made, a hush settled over the room. Within minutes, the obstetrician delivered a tiny premature infant and said, "OK, we have a pretty sick little baby here." The baby was limp, blue with no cry effort. He handed me the baby, just as the neonatologist raced into the room. The baby's heart rate was 80 with no respiratory effort and no muscle tone. We intubated and performed chest compressions; he responded so we quickly stabilized him and moved him to the NICU.

As the hours unfolded, we learned more about the mother's history. She was a prostitute and drug addict and had received no prenatal care. This was her second pregnancy. The other child had been removed from her and was in the custody of the local child protective services group—HRS.

The baby was delivered at 27 weeks' gestation and was diagnosed with Duboztiz Syndrome (a disfiguring condition). Over the ensuing weeks, his condition became worse. If there was a complication of prematurity, he seemed to get it. He had profound respiratory distress syndrome (RDS) requiring prolonged intubation and ventilation, he had collapsed lungs with bilateral chest tubes. He had a rash that required treatment for 21 days. He had a grade III intraventricular hemorrhage. The list of complications were lengthy as this little guy struggled to survive.

The baby's mother saw him only once when she was wheeled from the recovery room to the postpartum unit the day he was born. She left the hospital as soon as she could. She never gave him a name. She did call once when he was a few days old, but after that there was no contact from her or any other family member. This baby was totally alone in this world of horror.

Over a period of time, the seriousness of the situation began to "sink in" with the nursing staff. We watched this baby's daily struggle to live, watched him endure procedures and interventions without someone coming to see him to let him know he was loved. He was without a soul in this world to care about him. More than once I stood at his bedside and, to myself, questioned our continued efforts to pull him back, once again, from the brink of death. What were we saving him for? With all these serious complications, how could he ever be "normal"? Who would ever want to adopt a baby with his problems? If he lived, would he spend his life going from one foster care home to the next?

But, despite my questions and philosophical quandaries, the little guy became important to us. We found ourselves falling in love with him. He had a real bad habit of "trying to die" on night shift. Several times at four o'clock in the morning, he stopped breathing and had to be resuscitated (coded). The night nurses decided, after a few weeks, that he needed a name and they started calling him "Cody," because he had coded so many times on them. And so it was, he became Cody.

Slowly he progressed. At about 4 months of age, Cody was big enough for a crib even though he was still on oxygen with all the complications that entails: difficulty feeding, difficulty breathing, diffi-culty gaining weight. But he was one tough little soldier.

Then one day a miracle happened. I thought the miracle had been his survival, but I had a lot to learn. Our social worker contacted HRS and learned that Cody had a brother who was in foster care with a cou-ple who were adopting him. After conversations with the foster parents, they agreed to "meet" Cody with no promises and no commitments.

Once again, the nursing staff faced a dilemma. We overwhelmingly felt they should be made fully aware of Cody's long-term prognosis, which was not all that great. Had they been told about his mother's activities while pregnant with Cody? And did they understand what tak-ing this very special child would mean?

The big day arrived. Tammy, the adoptive mother, came to the unit, and what followed left an indelible impression on us all. We were wit-nesses to the amazing power of love. Tammy took one long look at Cody and simply said, "Oh isn't he beautiful? We just have to take this baby!" And there you have it. The miracle of miracles—love so sweet and pure that it transcended the problems and wires and words and prognoses. She took Cody up on her ample bosom and rocked him and sang softly to him, and he became the luckiest little boy.

Tammy and Stan (the father) became part of our unit. Daily they came and learned about Cody's complex care—such as the medica-tions, monitors, oxygen, feedings, routines, and need for follow-up appointments (of which there were many), but most importantly they came to love this little boy and to give him a chance that we could not have dreamed possible.

Tammy liked the name Cody and decided to keep it. The other nurses and I looked at one another with trepidation and wondered if we should tell her how he got the name. Eventually someone did tell her, and she laughed the jolly laugh we had come to love.

At 5 months of age, Cody was discharged home to Tammy and Stan. It was not an easy journey, but they held true to their faith in God and their love and commitment to this little boy.

Today Cody is 8 years old and is an active, happy, sweet little boy. He has been officially adopted by Tammy and Stan. Over the years, Tammy has given us updates on his progress. She came to see us over the holidays and brought pictures that warmed my heart and brought tears to my eyes for he was a happy, radiant little boy, looking normal, living, growing, and thriving in this home of love. Cody still has problems, but Tammy does not dwell on them. She accentuates the positive and takes them all in stride.

And I marvel, as a healthcare professional constantly facing ethical issues of life and death, and "quality of life," and whether to resuscitate or not, that we are not "in charge" of these domains, merely stewards of knowledge, experience, and expertise. Caring for Cody changed me as a nurse by broadening my perspective of what we do every day, and deepened my conviction that our work with these babies and families impacts lives for a very long time. Cody's survival is an example of the extraordinary advances in medicine and nursing. Now I know that my part is to do my job very well, dispense care, support families, and do all that I can to send these babies out into the world in the best possible shape and never underestimate the power of love.

BARGAINING THAT PAYS OFF
by Leokadia Bryk (Florida, USA)

Some people can look very ordinary, like a man in his 30s wearing a baseball cap who is casually dressed in shorts, shirt, and sneakers sitting down and writing a personal check. But behind ordinary looks can be a very extraordinary story.

This man was married with two children. He experienced a traumatic closed-head injury following an impulsive jump out of the moving car his wife was driving. His action was the result of hearing from his wife that she planned to divorce him. This young man was referred to our psychiatric department 2 months after the injury.

Psychiatric nursing includes caring for people who are in emotional and psychological pain. Unlike medical-surgical nursing where certain signs indicate physical pain, emotional pain is harder to detect. Besides the effects of the head trauma, this man was also experiencing emotional pain. His pain was acutely felt by all the staff. He was gaunt and disheveled, with a pained expression on his face most of the time. He yelled, whined, and cried almost constantly. Due to the head injury, he had frequent restlessness and irritability spells. He required intense help with toileting, feeding, cleaning, ambulating, and hydration. Mr. P was unable to remain in a geri chair even with a tabletop for too long. He would slide under the table or raise his legs over it. We tried using the "merry walker" so he could walk or sit. Unfortunately, he would climb under or over and that left him still at high-risk for falls. As much as we did not like to do so, we had to restrain his wrists and ankles to prevent injury. Of course, this intensified his restlessness, and medication did not seem to reduce his agitation.

We couldn't just ignore these situations. It pained the staff as much as the patient. We understood how frustrating it was for him. The staff members were feeling the strain and eventually it created a drain on emotional reserves. The charge nurse at one point started crying because of the stress. She was responsible for 15 other patients. This man required three staff persons at all times to transfer him from and to the chair/bed/bathroom due to his impulsiveness. When he ambulated, it was like a dog straining on a leash. Each transfer required removal of and reapplication of the restraints. My role was mainly supervisory, but my office was on the same floor so I was acutely aware of the situation.

One day one of the activity therapists approached me, frustrated, saying, "Can't we use a different restraint? He's starting to get sores from these restraints. What about a vest posey?" Sadly I had to remind her of the ban on vest poseys because of potential strangulation. My response did not deter this young woman who was advocating for this man. Each question of why and how felt like a "push" until I delivered a new idea. Like a snapshot, I visualized a diaper restraint. Yes, yes it could work! I was so excited I shared the idea. Together with her, another activity therapist, and I, we developed a crude primitive restraint out of a blanket. We tried it and it worked! He had no wrist and ankle restraints and the new restraint kept him from climbing out. It was success #1.

One of Mr. P's problems was communication. He was unable to present a coherent message. He seemed to have expressive aphasia. One day I found him whining with a pained look on his face. It is so hard to communicate comfort, to share soothing words that could ease some pain with a patient when you do not understand what they want. He mentioned his wife, and I, being the optimist, believed he was trying to express some concern about her (she did visit on a regular basis). I responded as if I understood him, telling him his wife was okay. He calmed down. I think he understood.

Another challenge while caring for him was the waning motivation and energy levels of the staff. I became more and more conscious of this situation, hearing and seeing the struggles they encountered with Mr. P. This was a double challenge since budget is always uppermost in the many decisions I must make. But I felt compassion for them and ventured to ask my director if we could assign one person to the patient, thus giving some respite to the technicians. This strategy had a calming effect for Mr. P, since someone was giving him constant attention. Unbeknownst to me, having one person care for him was the first stage of treatment at the rehabilitation institute where he was transferred. But in Mr. P's case, it took two persons to care for him. We had gotten to the point where the technicians, while doing their 15-minute checks, would wheel him in the geri chair with them around the unit.

The ultimate challenge and always uppermost in our minds was discharge planning. We were attentive to length of stay and wanted a meaningful placement for him. The charge nurse of the unit, having had previous experience with head-injured people, sensed Mr. P had a rehabilitation potential. Our medical director concurred with this possibility. We knew that 2 months post-head injury is not the best time to determine the full outcome of a patient's recovery potential. But the staff, charge nurse, utilization review nurse, and discharge planner had to tangle with the insurance company daily about his placement. The insurance company insisted a nursing home was his only option. However, the charge nurse had to give nurse-to-nurse reports up to 3 times a day. A nursing home would not be able to provide the kind of care he needed. Because of her insistence, different options were pursued. The insurance company kept balking at the requirement for physical and occupational therapies. The charge nurse felt he would vegetate in a nursing home. Finally, a neurologist rehabilitation institute was found where he could qualify. It took a few weeks of battling before a satisfying outcome was reached. All of the team members had minor skirmishes with the insurance company, but these were overcome one by one. I have never seen such strong patient advocacy in my entire nursing career.

This is a story with a marvelous ending. The marketing director of the rehabilitation institute kept in close contact with the charge nurse before and after discharge. The charge nurse received an invitation to the institute and asked me to accompany her. I was eager to see the program. I've always enjoyed follow-ups, finding out how a patient responded to treatment. So we visited the institute and found our Mr. P sitting calmly, dressed casually, learning how to write a check. When he rose to greet us, no unsteadiness was detected, and he was able to speak clearly and distinctly. Saying to the charge nurse as clear as a bell, "If it weren't for you, I wouldn't be here."

TAKING THE TIME TO SEE SUBTLE CHANGES
by Kathleen Young (Florida, USA)

Even as a fledgling nurse, I tried to look at people as "whole" and not the "sum of their parts." Triage is not considered the favorite assignment of most emergency department nurses. Although I would not want a steady diet of triage, I see it as a place where I can use my assessment and interviewing skills to evaluate each patient, plan care based on my observations, and implement care by appropriately assigning each person to the right area and to the right level of acuity or priority. At the end of most shifts when I have been the triage nurse, I have checked with the care providers to evaluate my decision-making and ultimately to see how the patients have done. The entire nursing process starts with the decisions made by the triage nurse.

One evening, Mrs. X walked into the triage area with a big smile and a slight limp. She was in her mid-30s. Her chief complaint was "my leg hurts." She continued to smile and giggle every so often throughout my questions. I began my physical assessment while I asked her questions. I watched how she moved, spoke, and breathed during the interview. Had she been injured recently? "No, just up on a ladder fixing the roof."

No falls, missteps, or bumps that she remembered. I assessed her pulse, temperature, and movement in each lower extremity. Everything was normal. I checked for a Homan's sign, which might indicate a blood clot, and it was positive on the painful leg.

The hunt for risk factors was on. The risk factors for thromboembolic problems are immobility, which didn't seem to fit a young woman who was fixing her roof. She denied a history of cancer, recent trauma, or surgery. Being female and hormone therapy, which includes birth control medications, is another risk factor. When I asked her about birth control, she laughed loudly and said, "Who has sex?"

Before I could ask her for her last menstrual period to assess the possibility of pregnancy, her sister playfully hit her on the shoulder saying, "Don't you remember? You had your tubes tied." Then the sister said, "You have been so forgetful recently. I worry about you." Although said playfully, I could tell that this had not been Mrs. X's first episode of forgetfulness, and her sister was genuinely concerned. This raised a red flag for me because I had never met a woman who forgot about not having to worry about contraception.

My attentions turned to assessing her neurological status … after all, it wasn't just "the leg pain" anymore. She was Mrs. X, a woman with leg pain, inappropriate laughter that I had first attributed to nervousness (now I wasn't quite so sure), a positive Homan's sign, and forgetfulness. Intuitively, I knew there was more than a leg problem. I assessed her cranial nerves, which required her to stick out her tongue, move it from side to side, show me her teeth, and other amusing maneuvers. She laughed when asked to do each maneuver, but complied. I noted her pupils responded unequally and at different speeds. Her grips, arm and leg strengths were also assessed, and there were subtle differences.

Mrs. X's vital signs were within normal limits, and she showed no signs of drooling, facial droop, or other conditions that would make me think of a cerebrovascular accident (CVA). I gave Mrs. X a "3" priority or a non-urgent assignment and sent her to the emergency department (ED). However, I kept a close eye on her and called the charge nurse in the back room. I told her I was sure something else was going on with Mrs. X. I was told Mrs. X would be called soon, and she was.

I finished my shift as triage nurse and walked to the back. I noted a grossly abnormal head scan on the x-ray view box. I saw the neurosurgeon leaving one of the rooms and checked the patient board. He was leaving Mrs. X's room. Her CT was the one on the view box. It showed a large, menacing mass—a global meningioma.

I took a deep breath and walked into Mrs. X's room where I saw three teary-eyed people and Mrs. X, who was smiling. She put her hands out, I took them, and she gave me a big hug. She motioned to the young man and said, "Honey, this is the nurse who found I had cancer." I was taken aback by her cheerfulness, but reminded myself that this had been part of her earlier behavior. Her husband shook my hand and mouthed, "Thank you." I met her parents, who, although shaken, expressed their thanks also. I hadn't really "found" her cancer but had gotten the ball rolling toward her diagnosis. It would have been so easy for her to have slipped through the cracks. I told Mrs. X and her family I would keep them in my thoughts and prayers.

I checked out of the ED and went to my car. I sat there for awhile pondering the events of the evening. A young, active woman had walked into an emergency department for her leg pain only to find out she had a brain tumor. Mrs. X probably did not appreciate fully the seriousness of the situation, but her life had certainly changed forever in just a few short hours. Mrs. X was transferred the next day to a university medical center. Although I tried, I was not able to find out what happened after her transfer.

I was thankful I had the skills and experience to evaluate her not as a "leg pain," but as a person with leg pain ... a whole person. I was thankful I listened to what she said and didn't say and had taken the time to look at the subtle changes. Each nursing experience I have helps me grow as a nurse, and I integrate each of those experiences into my practice. I was thankful the clues to her underlying condition were there and I discovered their importance. Most of all, I was glad that I was the triage nurse that night.

The greatness of nurse work permeates each and every story of this chapter. The settings are eclectic, but the underlying theme of doing more than is expected is clearly evident.

We have read about nurses who make the impossible happen and do it because they care enough and believe.

We have read about nurses who helped change the laws and the way the system operates so the family can benefit; nurses who expressed words that are difficult to say and difficult to hear but let the truth be known for the sake of the family; nurses who were members of dedicated teams and groups of caretakers working the same goal, the same vision, and the same dream. The value of nurses to the healthcare team, the importance of their work to the families, and the endless dedication to what is good and what is right are the expressions in the stories of this chapter.

Above all, nurses are witnesses to prevailing transformations often beyond our control. Transformations caused by fate, human connections, discipline, and belief in a higher power are all done in the spirit of serving others.

(Special thanks to the Florida Nurses Association, Willa Fuller, Amanda Flenghi, Dr. Francis Smith, Dr. Pat Quigley, & Paula Massey and the incredible authors of "Clinical Exemplars" who encourage nurses to share their stories.)

AFTERWORD

Closure

These hands have helped heal and hold, So many patients, young and old, So many people, shy and bold, So many seasons, hot and cold. The touch of a nurse's hand is as precious as gold.

—Jennifer McElligott Carley (New York, USA)

Dear reader:

Have you ever asked yourself, why nursing? Have you ever sat back and reflected on the greatness in the profession of nursing? What is it that makes people choose nursing for a career? What piques a nurse's interest, fuels her desire, or captivates her mind? I have a few ideas that came from years of reading nurses' stories.

It is the hands. It is the hands that touch the dying patient and wipe away the tears. It is knowing hands. Hands that perform CPR compressions, deliver medications for pain, and monitor every respiration. It is hands that are ready to hold, nourish, and comfort that make all the difference in the world.

It is the hands, the fingers, that manipulate the tiniest of toes. It is the fingers that feel a fleeting pulse or warm an aching joint. It is the fingers that time birthing contractions and cradle the infant's precious head.

It is the hands that gently care for the child post-op and teach a mother to bathe a 5-pound baby or to give insulin to a teenager. It is the hands that oh-so-carefully touch liquid to the parched lips of the dying man. It is the hands that stroke a patient's forehead when the seizure is over, and the hands that drip life-saving medication into a needy vein. It is these hands that tenderly wield high-tech tools and instruments, and the hands in prayer at the bedside. Whoever you are, dear nurse, it is your hands that make life better.

It is the heart. It is clear in these stories that most nurses become nurses because of a heartfelt, caring spirit. The ability to help those in need without a second thought, without a shadow of a doubt, is nursing. It is the great nurses who continually give above and beyond, who go the extra mile. It is these nurses who truly comprise the "heart of nursing." This desire to care about others in the local and global community keeps our profession great and strong.

It is the mind. Nurses have incredible minds. Their educational preparation has provided them with critical thinking skills and astute decision-making abilities. Science and psychosocial information has provided a foundation for nursing knowledge. Ethics, psychology, philosophy are woven into the curriculum. Pathophysiology courses and nursing care modalities prepare the nurse for a variety of patient problems. Medication administration is impossible without the ability to solve complex mathematical problems. Tedious analysis of normal and abnormal laboratory data and endless pharmacology courses prepare the nurse to administer literally hundreds of drugs each week. These challenges stretch the mind, but they ultimately allow the nurse to deliver safe nursing care.

It is a calling. Nurses know it, but their style is not to show it. Nurses are the heroes of healthcare, not in the forefront but omnipresent. They are the silent partners behind the scenes. Each nurse knows the meaning of her or his work. Each nurse knows the feeling that good care brings—the feeling of "making a difference."

Transforming care is what it really is. Nurses are transforming lives, transforming healthcare, and transforming the profession each day. Nursing is care that goes beyond the norm because it includes advocating, reassuring, and preventing illness. The performance is thorough, scientific, and exact. Nurses know what is supposed to be done, and they get it done.

Nurses make it happen. They often save lives. At the very least, they make life a little better for the remaining time a patient has. Nurses have an incredible impact on patients. Unlike almost any other profession, nurses and patients frequently keep in touch long after their encounters. Families, also, become friends. Nurses name their children after patients. The families never forget. The nurses certainly never forget. It is human connection that is meaningful to patients and the families, and this, in itself, is so unique to nursing.

It is the caring for sure, but the ordinary flow of real life cannot be discounted in the stories presented in this book. I began this book with a story about nurses in long-term care. It was a story about a song bird—and the nurses who purchased the songbird—that sang so sweetly as the patient took his last breath. The stories in this book reveal fantastic accounts of skill, devotion, respect, and promise. There are stories that define the essence of nursing, that communicate wisdom, spirituality, and love. There are also narratives about comfort, compassion, cultural competence, and courage. There are even those that illustrate how nurses handle crisis and manage death experiences. All the stories have a consistent bond—allegiance and loyalty to patients and their families.

It is my hope that in reading the stories of nurses, the sweet moments and tender giving, you will recognize the work of nurses. You will indeed see that nurses truly make a difference. It is my desire that the genuine goodness of nurses be brought from behind the scenes to the forefront for all to see and celebrate.

The intention of this book is to give credit to nurses who have made a difference in the lives of patients. It is to say thanks, in a very big way, to nurses who might feel ordinary but who are truly extraordinary.

Let us all recognize that nurses see what no one else sees, hear what no one else hears, and feel what no one else feels. In the wee hours of the morning, it is the nurse who provides life-saving actions. Yet, another nurse colleague in another part of the world may be doing exactly the same thing, serving another, or breathing life into one who cannot do it alone.

Nurses are privileged to see healing and witness firsthand the remarkable world of nursing. Now you have witnessed the gifts nurses bring to many. Now you are filled up by the stories of nurses who have left a heritage of caring that will be marked in time. Like a string of pearls, these stories are handed down to you.

The tradition of nursing is rich in historical and present knowledge. Nurses are proud of their work, proud to be nurses. This book records the history of nursing past, present, and future. May you always be comforted by knowing that a nurse is close by should the need arise.

Sincerely,
Sharon Hudacek

Books Published by the Honor Society of Nursing, Sigma Theta Tau International

A Daybook for Nurses: Making a Difference Each Day, Hudacek, 2004.

The Adventurous Years: Leaders in Action 1973-1999, Henderson, 1998.

As We See Ourselves: Jewish Women in Nursing, Benson, 2001.

Building and Managing a Career in Nursing: Strategies for Advancing Your Caree Miller, 2003.

Cadet Nurse Stories: The Call for and Response of Women During World War I Perry and Robinson, 2001.

Collaboration for the Promotion of Nursing, Briggs, Merk, and Mitchell, 2003.

Creating Responsive Solutions to Healthcare Change, McCullough, 2001.

Gerontological Nursing Issues for the 21st Century, Gueldner and Poon, 1999.

The HeART of Nursing: Expressions of Creative Art in Nursing, Wendler, 2002.

The Image Editors: Mind, Spirit, and Voice, Hamilton, 1997.

Immigrant Women and Their Health: An Olive Paper, Ibrahim Meleis, Lipson Muecke and Smith, 1998.

The Language of Nursing Theory and Metatheory, King and Fawcett, 1997.

Making a Difference: Stories from the Point of Care, Hudacek, 2000.

Making a Difference: Stories from the Point of Care, Volume 2, Hudacek, 2004.

The Neuman Systems Model and Nursing Education: Teaching Strategies an Outcomes, Lowry, 1998.

Nurses' Moral Practice: Investing and Discounting Self, Kelly, 2000.

Nursing and Philanthropy: An Energizing Metaphor for the 21st Century, McBride 2000.

Ordinary People, Extraordinary Lives: The Stories of Nurses, Smeltzer and Vlasses 2003.

Pivotal Moments in Nursing Leaders Who Changed the Path of a Profession, House and Player, 2004.

The Roy Adaptation Model-Based Research: 25 Years of Contributions to Nursin Science, Boston Based Adaptation Research in Nursing Society, 1999.

Stories of Family Caregiving: Reconsideration of Theory, Literature, and Life, Poirie and Ayres, 2002.

Virginia Avenel Henderson: Signature for Nursing, Hermann, 1997.

For more information and to order these books from the Honor Society of Nursing, Sigm Theta Tau International, visit the society's Web site at www.nursingsociety.org/publications , o go to www.nursingknowledge.org/stti/books, the Web site of Nursing Knowledg International, the honor society's sales and distribution division, or call 1.888.NKI.4.YOU (U.S and Canada) or +1.317.634.8171 (Outside U.S. and Canada).